The International Library c

T0227810

MENTAL HEALTH AND INFANT DEVELOPMENT

VOLUME ONE

Founded by C. K. Ogden

The International Library of Psychology

DEVELOPMENTAL PSYCHOLOGY
In 32 Volumes

MENTAL HEALTH AND INFANT DEVELOPMENT

Proceedings of the International Seminar held by the World Federation for Mental Health at Chichester, England

Volume One: Papers and Discussions

Edited by KENNETH SODDY

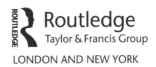

Routledge
Taylor & Francis Group

LONDON AND NEW YORK

First published in 1956
by Routledge
2 Park Square, Milton Park, Abingdon, Oxfordshire OX14 4RN
711 Third Avenue, New York, NY 10017

First issued in paperback 2014

Routledge is an imprint of the Taylor and Francis Group, an informa business

British Library Cataloguing in Publication Data
A CIP catalogue record for this book
is available from the British Library

Mental Health and Infant Development
ISBN 0415-21007-0
Developmental Psychology: 32 Volumes
ISBN 0415-21128-X
The International Library of Psychology: 204 Volumes
ISBN 0415-19132-7

ISBN 13: 978-1-138-87515-9 (pbk)
ISBN 13: 978-0-415-21007-2 (hbk)

CONTENTS

CONTENTS

Part Three

STUDIES OF INFANT RELATIONSHIP FORMATION

Part Four

DIFFERENT CULTURAL PATTERNS AND TECHNOLOGICAL CHANGE

CONTENTS

Part Five

SOCIAL AND COMMUNITY PROVISIONS FOR MENTAL HYGIENE

Part Six

TECHNIQUES FOR CHANGING SOCIAL PRACTICES

Part Seven

STUDIES IN PSYCHOLOGY AND NEUROLOGY, AND AIDS TO EDUCATION

Part Eight

PREFACE

THE PRESENT VOLUME, together with its accompanying volume of Case Histories, constitutes the proceedings of the Seminar on Mental Health and Infant Development held at Bishop Otter Training College, Chichester, Sussex, England, from July 19th to August 10th, 1952. The Seminar was organized by the World Federation for Mental Health with support from the World Health Organization and a number of other organizations to which acknowledgments are gratefully given on another page. The present volume includes all the lectures given at the Seminar, presented in a reduced form in order to keep the size of the volume within reasonable proportions; and an account of its general structure and functioning. Volume II contains approximately one half of the case material specially prepared for use at the Seminar. Reference to the cases in Volume II will be found scattered throughout the text of Volume I, and in addition there are numerous references to other cases discussed at the Seminar for which it has not been possible to find room in the selection printed. It is hoped that occasional reference to these unpublished cases will not constitute a source of difficulty to readers, but it was deemed wiser to keep such references in the text so that readers could judge the extent to which lectures were based on present day clinical experience. Numerals in brackets throughout the text refer to the Bibliography at the end of the volume.

ACKNOWLEDGMENTS

A GREAT NUMBER of people were involved in planning, and in other ways making it possible to hold the Seminar; and in distinguishing some names for mention here, I should like to convey the warm thanks of the World Federation for Mental Health to all those who helped in the common task.

Perhaps the real originators of the Seminar were Dr. Frank Fremont-Smith of the Josiah Macy, Jr. Foundation, New York, and Dr. J. R. Rees, Director of the Federation, who planned the International Preparatory Commission preceding the International Congress on Mental Health, London, 1948, which, under the chairmanship of the late Dr. Harry Stack Sullivan, created the atmosphere which made future developments possible. Their help, throughout, was a constant source of inspiration.

At the meeting of the Inter-Professional Advisory Committee of the Federation in Dublin, 1951, and subsequently in London, Paris, Leeds, New York and Mexico City, many discussions were held involving, among others, Dr. Jenny Aubry (then Dr. Jenny Roudinesco), Dr. John Bowlby, Dr. Gerald Caplan, Prof. Bingham Dai, Dr. Henry Dicks, Mr. Lawrence K. Frank, Prof. Max Gluckman, Dr. G. R. Hargreaves, Dr. Madeleine Kerr, Prof. Olof Kinberg, Prof. Otto Klineberg, Prof. Jaap Koekebakker, Dr. Cyrille Koupernik, Prof. Daniel Lagache, Prof. William Line, Prof. D. R. MacCalman, Dr. Margaret Mead, Prof. G. P. Meredith, Mme. Rhoda Métraux, Mrs. Grace O'Neill, Dr. Yves Porc'her, Dr. J. R. Rees, Prof. T. Ferguson Rodger, Prof. T. S. Simey, Dr. Frank Fremont-Smith, Miss Helen Speyer, Dr. René Spitz, Dr. George S. Stevenson, Dr. Pierre Turquet, and Dr. René Zazzo.

In addition, as Director of the Seminar, I visited nearly all the institutions which co-operated in the Seminar. A list of these is given, and full acknowledgments are made, in Volume II, which contains the Case Histories.

However, the Seminar needed more than ideas, and many friends helped in securing the necessary financial support. The decision which made the Seminar possible was the willingness of the Regional Office for Europe to incorporate it within a series of inter-country activities financed by the World Health Organization, in Europe. The Regional Office arranged for the attendance of thirty-five participants from countries in Europe and also contributed about $10,000 U.S. towards the organizational costs. For this decision and for a very great deal of practical help which accompanied it, we are particularly indebted to Dr. N. D. Begg, Director of the Regional Office for Europe, to Dr. G. R. Hargreaves, Chief of the Mental Health Section of WHO, and to Dr. Kjellberg and several other members of the Regional Office staff.

Other WHO Regions also co-operated and arranged for the attendance of thirteen participants from regions other than Europe.

Financial support was forthcoming from other sources, and we gratefully acknowledge a subvention of $3,500 from UNESCO, and the help of Dr. W. D. Wall of the Department of Education. Through the good offices of Dr. Margaret Mead, Dr. Fremont-Smith and Mr. Lawrence K. Frank, a grant of $15,000 from the United States National Advisory Mental Health Council (U.S. Public Health Service) was given, for our use, to the Society for Applied Anthropology for the preparation of case material, including a proportion of the costs of the present volumes; and $6,750 from the Grant Foundation of New York for the travel and maintenance costs of the American members of the teaching Faculty. To Prof. Robert Debré and his colleagues we tender our thanks for a grant of $831 from the Centre International de l'Enfance, in Paris, for the costs of one member of the teaching Faculty and one participant from France Outre-mer. The Federation itself bore the costs of two British participants.

Among our many other willing helpers, we must especially thank all those who did the practical work in preparation of the material, in attending as members of the Faculty and in joining the Seminar as participants. To our great regret, Dr. Sybille Escalona, then of the Menninger Foundation, Topeka, Kansas, U.S.A., was prevented from joining the Faculty by a last minute illness. Dr. Edith Jackson, of Yale University, nobly filled her place at very short notice. The names of all who helped us by their presence are recorded in the appropriate place, but special mention should be made of Miss Judith Jackson, the Administrator of the Seminar. Miss Jackson successfully brought her great experience and personal charm to the task of making a very heterogeneous family happy and putting them in a frame of mind to give of their best to the Seminar.

To the Principal and staff of Bishop Otter College, in particular Miss A. M. Reed and Mr. H. Bell, our great appreciation is also due for making us so comfortable and welcome; and to the Rt. Rev. the Lord Bishop of Chichester, His Worship the Mayor of Chichester, Dr. Joshua Carse and the Chairman, Committee and Staff of Graylingwell Hospital for their hospitality. It was gratifying also to have as a visitor, the British Minister of Health, the Rt. Hon. Iain Macleod, M.P., and we should like to thank Sir Weldon Dalrymple Champneys, Bart., Deputy Chief Medical Officer, Ministry of Health, for welcoming the foreign visitors so gracefully, and in so many languages, on behalf of the British Government.

Finally, to our own office staff our grateful thanks, and in particular to Miss Esther Thornton, Secretary-General of WFMH, for her constant support and help in planning and carrying out the Seminar, and in editing the Proceedings.

KENNETH SODDY, M.D.,
Director of the Seminar.
Assistant Director, World Federation for Mental Health.

LIST OF MEMBERS

MARGARET ADAMS, U.S.A. (Member of Faculty)
Director, Programme of Graduate Study in Paediatric Nursing, Teachers' College, Columbia University, New York City.

BELINDE AFTALION, Spain
Hospital del Rey, Madrid.

JOYCE M. AKESTER, U.K. (Member of Faculty)
Superintendent Nursing Officer, Health Department, West Sussex County Council, Chichester.

CHARIKLIA ALEXANDRAKI, Greece
Child Welfare Adviser, Ministère de la Prévoyance et de la Santé Publique, Athènes.

PER ANCHERSEN, Norway
Assistant Professor at Psychiatric Clinic, University of Oslo.

JENNY AUBRY (Jenny Roudinesco), France (Member of Faculty)
Médecin de la Policlinique de l'Hôpital Bichat, Paris.

JACOBUS P. BOEKHOLD, Netherlands
Paediatrician in charge of Child Hygiene, Department of Zuid-Holland. Director of a day-nursery for convalescent children. Child Guidance Clinic, Leiden.

HELVI BOOTHE, U.S.A. (Member of Faculty)
Director of Psychiatric Social Work, The Menninger Foundation, Topeka, Kansas.

MARJAN BORSTNAR, Yugoslavia
Chief of Department, Mental Hospital, Ljubljana. Physician, Ljubljana Polyclinic, Psycho-hygienic Consultation Centre.

JULIETTE FAVEZ-BOUTONIER, France (Member of Faculty)
Professeur de Psychologie, Université de Strasbourg.

JOHN BOWLBY, U.K. (Visiting member of Faculty)
Medical Director, Children's Department, Tavistock Clinic, London.

JEANNE BROYELLE, France
Médecin Inspecteur de la Santé. Médecin Chef de la Protection maternelle et infantile de la Seine, Paris.

PAULETTE CAHN, France
Attachée de Recherches au Centre national de Recherche scientifique et Centre psychopédagogique, Strasbourg.

MARIE-TH. CALLEWAERT, Belgium
Neuro-psychiatre infantile. Membre du Comité directeur de la Ligue nationale belge d'Hygiène mentale, Bruxelles.

BALTAZAR CARAVEDO, Jr., Peru
Chief of Child Guidance Clinic, Ministry of Public Health, Lima.

MICHEL CATSANIS, Greece
Médecin Neuro-Psychiatre, Athènes.

ANDRE CHAURAND, France
Médecin Directeur de l'Institut pédotechnique (Centre d'Observation et Ecole de Formation de Rééducateurs), Toulouse.

MARGUERITE CLAVEAU, France
Directeur Départemental de la Santé de la Moselle, Metz.

ADDA CORTI, Italy
Psychologue auprès du Centre médico-pédagogique de l'ONMI de Rome.

SIMONNE M. A. COTTE, France
Assistante Principale de l'Hygiène Mentale Départementale des Bouches du Rhône. Psychologue expert près le Tribunal des Mineurs délinquents. Comité Enfance Déficiente, Marseille.

PIERRE L. V. A. DEMOULIN, Belgium
Médecin Inspecteur des établissements pour malades mentaux et enfants anormaux, Ministère de la Santé publique, Bruxelles.

JOSE DIAZ, Mexico
Head of Department of Mental Hygiene, General Maximino Avila Camacho Maternal and Child Welfare Centre, Mexico City.

LORIMER DODS, Australia
Director of Institute of Child Welfare, University of Sydney.

MIRIAM FLORENTIN, U.K. (Member of Faculty)
Senior Assistant Medical Officer of Health, County Borough of West Ham, Essex.

ANNA FREUD, U.K. (Visiting Member of Faculty)
Psychoanalyst, Hampstead Nursery, London.

RITA FULDA, Germany
Public Health Officer engaged on mass survey and examination of school children, Bonn.

ANNA B. GARDINER, U.K.
Senior Assistant Medical Officer, Kent County Council, Maidstone.

MARIJA GAJIC, Yugoslavia
Adviser to the Council of Public Health and Social Welfare of Yugoslavia, Belgrade.

MARCELLE GEBER, France
Médecin Psychologue. Attachée de Consultation d'Hygiène mentale de la Policlinique de l'Hôpital Bichat. Médecin consultant au Centre d'Hygiène Mentale de Soissons.

SOPHIE GEDEON, Greece
Membre du Conseil Supérieur de l'Education au Ministère de l'Education et Professeur de Psychologie et d'Hygiène Mentale a l'Ecole pour Assistantes Sociales d'UWCA, Athènes.

SABRY GIRGIS, Egypt
Director of Neuropsychiatric Clinic, School Health Department, Cairo. Lecturer in Child Psychiatry and Mental Health, Cairo School of Social Work.

ERNST GJORUP, Denmark
Chief Physician, Norre Hospital. Head of Child Guidance Clinic and Paediatrician at institutions in Copenhagen.

N. V. GOPALASWAMI, India
Professor of Psychology, University of Mysore. Director of Nursery-Infant Schools, Mysore.

ANN A. GRAHAM, U.K.
Superintendent Health Visitor, Northumberland County Council Health Department, Newcastle-on-Tyne.

WILHELM K. HAGEN, Germany
Head of Section of Public Health, Child Health and Welfare, Health Education and Anti-Tuberculosis Work, Ministry of the Interior, Bonn. Member of Board of Directors of the 'Deutsches Gesundheitsmuseum.'

PER HEGRENAES, Norway
Board of Health Medical Officer (psychiatrist). Consultant psychiatrist at the Municipal Hospital, and Police Medical Officer, Trondheim.

BARTHOLD HENGEVELD, Netherlands
Paediatrician. Director Open-Air Day-Nursery for delicate and convalescent children, Arnhem. Medical officer for child hygiene in Gelderland.

RENE HENNY, Switzerland
Médecin á l'Office médico-pédagogique vaudois, Lausanne.

FERNANDO HENRIQUES, U.K. (Member of Faculty)
Lecturer in social anthropology, University of Leeds.

REINO T. HUTTUNEN, Finland
Consultant on Mental Hygiene, Public Health Demonstration and Teaching Area, Uusimaa, Helsinki.

EDITH JACKSON, U.S.A. (Member of Faculty)
Clinical Professor of Paediatrics and Psychiatry, Yale University School of Medicine.

ARNOLD G. JOSELIN, U.K. (Visiting Member of Faculty)
Lecturer, Department of Psychology, University of Leeds. Director of film 'Life Begins in Leeds'.

CYRILLE KOUPERNIK, France (Member of Faculty)
Pédiatre et psychiatre infantile, Hôpital des Enfants-Malades, Paris. Centre International de l'Enfance, Paris.

HARALD KREUTZFELDT, Denmark
Medical Officer, Board of Health, Copenhagen.

DOLORES G. LA CARO, U.S.A. (Puerto Rico)
Chief of Bureau, Medical Social Services. Director of Mental Hygiene Programme, Puerto Rico.

A. M. LAMONT, South Africa
Psychiatrist, Union of South Africa Department of Health, Mental Hygiene Branch, Pretoria.

EBBA LAURI, Finland
Field Supervisor of State School of Public Health Nursing. Instructor in Child Health, Helsinki.

IRENE LEZINE, France (Visiting Member of Faculty)
Psychologist, Laboratoire psycho-biologique de l'Enfant, Paris.

KARIN LUNDSTROM, Sweden
Councillor of Education, Board of Education, Stockholm.

D. R. MacCALMAN, U.K. (Member of Faculty)
Nuffield Professor of Psychiatry, University of Leeds.

ERNST MANSFELD, Germany
Public Health Officer, Stuttgart.

MARGARET MEAD, U.S.A. (Member of Faculty)
Assistant Curator of Anthropology, American Museum of Natural History, New York City.

G. P. MEREDITH, U.K. (Member of Faculty)
Professor of Psychology, University of Leeds.

LOUISE B. MESTEL, U.K. (Member of Faculty)
Lecturer, Department of Psychology, University of Leeds.

ALAN A. MONCRIEFF, U.K. (Visiting Member of Faculty)
Professor of Child Health, University of London.

W. MOSLEY, Canada
School of Hygiene, University of Toronto.

BIRGITTA NYRIN-BRENEL, Sweden
Paediatrician and Child Psychiatrist, Children's Hospital, Gothenburg.

YOSHIO OGAWA, Japan
Superintendent, Child Guidance Centre, Miyagi Prefecture, Sendai.

ELLI PAPATHEOPHILOU, Greece
Child Welfare Regional Supervisor, Ministère de Prévoyance Sociale et de la Santé Publique, Athènes.

LUIS E. PREGO, Uruguay
Child Psychiatrist. Technical Adviser on Mental Health, Department of Psychiatry, Children's Hospital, Montevideo.

EDUARDO QUINTERO MURO, Venezuela
Psychiatrist. Director of Mental Health Institute (Ministry of Health), Caracas.

JAMES ROBERTSON, U.K. (Visiting Member of Faculty)
Psychiatric Social Worker. Separation Research, Tavistock Clinic, London. Director of Film 'A Two-Year-Old Goes to Hospital.'

PHON SANGSINGKEO, Thailand
Director, Division of Hospitals for Mental Diseases, Ministry of Health, Bangkok.

MAGDALENE SCHIEK, Germany
Youth Welfare Official, German Protestant Church, Düsseldorf.

MOAMMER K. SHABENDER, Iraq
Medical Officer, Hospital for Mental and Nervous Diseases, Baghdad.

KENNETH SODDY, U.K. (Director of the Seminar)
Assistant Director, World Federation for Mental Health. Physician, Department of Psychological Medicine, University College Hospital, London. Psychiatrist, Child Guidance Training Centre, London.

ENCARNACION SOLER, Spain
Instructeur d'Hygiène publique á l'Ecole nationale de Puériculture, Madrid.

WALTER H. SPIEL, Austria
Secretary, Austrian League for Mental Health. Chief of Department of Child Psychiatry, University Clinic of Vienna.

xix

Part One

EDITOR'S INTRODUCTION

INTRODUCTION

THE SEMINAR on Mental Health and Infant Development held at Chichester from July 19th to August 10th, 1952, was, at that time, the first of its kind in which a number of people of different professional disciplines and from many countries were gathered together to study a specific aspect of the mental health field. In planning it, there were few precedents on which to proceed, but in fact, the Seminar was highly structured and had been built up in a series of inter-disciplinary, international discussions over a period of about two years. It took the form of a three weeks' residential training course in which fifty-one persons from thirty different countries were brought together, with a teaching staff of sixteen resident and seven visiting members, to learn about some of the phenomena of family life in the first two years of a baby.

The idea of such a Seminar was mooted in the Report of the International Preparatory Commission of the International Congress on Mental Health, London, 1948, which advocated the assembling of key people in inter-professional, international training courses. In April 1951, the Inter-Professional Advisory Committee of the World Federation for Mental Health met in Dublin to consider, among other things, the planning of permanent international institutes for research and training in mental health and, as a first step, suggested that experience could be gained by the organization of short-term training courses.

Due acknowledgment has been made on another page to those friends of the World Federation for Mental Health, including among their number private individuals and members of the staffs of Foundations, WHO, UNESCO and Government Agencies, who made this venture possible by their ideas, their personal interest and work, and by making money available. An immense amount of time and energy was willingly given by a great number of people to planning and collecting the necessary material; while a very heavy burden of responsibility and practical work was laid on the Executive Board of the Federation, its Director and staff.

THE PLAN OF WORK

The Seminar was based on a series of studies of actual children, used for teaching purposes by the highly qualified members of the Faculty. The participants were people of good professional

3

qualifications, holding influential positions in the Public Health and Child Welfare fields of their own countries. All who were present were subjected to an experience of international, mutual learning in the hope that, on return to their own work, they might have a wider horizon and enriched experience and, perhaps, a greater insight into the personal and cultural problems of the people among whom they work. At the same time there was the desire to conduct an experiment in an untried method of education, to seek some consensus of opinion on highly controversial matters and, indirectly, to improve the life of the child in his family.

Case material was collected from France, the United Kingdom and the United States—all countries in which work in this field had been in progress for many years. In the U.S.A. Dr. Margaret Mead and Mr. Lawrence K. Frank organized the collection of thirteen case studies from among existing research projects. These were presented in six groups and supported with carefully documented film records from the work of Dr. Mead herself, Professor Joseph Stone of Vassar College, Dr. Margaret Fries and Dr. René Spitz of New York. In France the collection of case material was under the supervision of Dr. Jenny Aubry (then Dr. Jenny Roudinesco), of Paris, with the co-operation of many others, on the general initiative of Dr. Yves Porc'her. Studies of parents undergoing a university training course, industrial artisans and rural workers were made in respect of their family life, and a special film on psychogenic retardation was compiled under Dr. Aubry's supervision. In the U.K., the preparation of material was under the supervision of Professor D. R. MacCalman, of the University of Leeds, and a new film showing the welfare background of the work, entitled *Life Begins in Leeds*, was made under the direction of Mr. Arnold Joselin. In addition, an inquiry was made into parental attitudes, by means of a questionnaire.

THE FACULTY

A complete list of all who took part in this Seminar can be found on page xv. In inviting members of the Faculty to take part, consideration was given first to profession and then to nationality. Having made a decision that British, French and American cases should be studied by participants coming mainly from Europe, it was decided to have a Faculty drawn from the three countries. Among the sixteen resident members of the Faculty, eight professional disciplines were represented including two anthropologists, four child psychiatrists, an educationalist, a paediatrician, three psychologists, a psychiatric social worker, two public health doctors (one of them being a psychiatrist in public health service), and two public health nurses. Visiting Faculty members included two child psychiatrists, a paediatrician, a non-medical psychoanalyst, three psychologists, and a psychiatric social worker. A paediatrician attended through the courtesy of the International Children's Centre of Paris.

THE PARTICIPANTS

The participants, except the two British and the French overseas representatives, were travelling on WHO short-term Fellowships, and responsibility for their selection lay with their respective governments. Naturally a guide was given to governments as to the type of person for whom the Seminar was intended, and it was stressed that senior people were wanted, who were responsible for organizing large departments or training programmes, and that all professional disciplines working in the child welfare field would be eligible. Sixteen European countries between them sent thirty-seven participants and the remaining fourteen came from other parts of the world, to make up fifty-one in all. A great deal of enthusiasm for the idea was shown by governments, and there was ample evidence of care in their interpretation of the wishes of the organizers.

Representatives from the following countries took part: Algeria, Australia, Austria, Belgium, Canada, Denmark, Egypt, Eire, Finland, France, Germany, Greece, India, Iraq, Italy, Japan, Mexico, the Netherlands, Norway, Peru, Spain, Sweden, Switzerland, Thailand, the Union of South Africa, the United Kingdom, the United States of America (Puerto Rico), Uruguay and Venezuela. The Algerian representative came at the expense of the International Children's Centre of Paris and the British participants at that of WFMH. There were twenty-two women and twenty-nine men.

Thirty-seven of the fifty-one were medically qualified, of whom twelve were practising psychiatrists, four psychiatrists in public health work, two in mental deficiency work, and one exclusively a child psychiatrist. Thirteen medical participants were public health officers, eight as medical officers of health and five as maternity and child welfare officers. Five were paediatricians in public service. Of the non-medical disciplines, five participants were psychologists, four social workers, one a psychiatric social worker, three public health nurses, and one an educationalist.

THE GENERAL ATMOSPHERE

The Seminar was held in a residential college which was well equipped, with spacious grounds and comfortable living accommodation. The social life of the Seminar was centred in the Federation Club, in which participants could entertain each other and their

5

friends. The work of the Seminar was enriched by the presence of a number of young children and in particular a one-year-old boy who, undesignedly, provided a practical demonstration of the capabilities of that age.

On the more technical side, the provision of an imaginative programme of visual aids, under the direction of Mr. Alan Staniland, with a library and an exhibition of propaganda material, gave valuable ideas to the participants.

It was clear that the participants came willingly, even eagerly, to the Seminar: but in a residential gathering of this kind, at which most of the participants are not experienced in cross-cultural contacts, something more is needed than general goodwill, if the experience is to be beneficial. The organizers were mindful of many examples of well-meant and well-conceived international gatherings which accomplished little, or even did harm, because of a failure to achieve mutual understanding and to provide each participant with a meaningful experience. At this Seminar the outstanding contribution was that of the Behavioural Sciences, in particular cultural anthropology and sociology, to the understanding of psychological and medical phenomena. It was, in addition, a source of strength to the Seminar that the teaching Faculty was composed of people who had taken a calculated risk in allowing their names to be identified with an experiment in a relatively unknown field. They were people who withstood the pressure of anxiety which so easily may arise in an international gathering of this type; and their leadership was characterized by permissiveness, adaptability, and a liberal professional knowledge.

THE PATTERN OF THE PROGRAMME

The programme consisted of lectures to the full Seminar followed by discussion, film projections and discussions, panel discussions, and five permanent working groups each of ten participants and three Faculty members (one group had eleven participants). These working groups undertook studies of the case material and discussions arising out of these.

In general, the day started with a lecture and question period lasting one hour and a quarter, followed by a group discussion period of about one and a half hours, and then a short film projection session. On each day, either the afternoon or the evening was left free, and in the time remaining for work, a two-hour session was devoted to a lecture or a full seminar discussion, group-reporting or panel discussion. Each working group had a discussion period nearly every day. There were eighteen days' work and every seventh day was completely free. All work was bilingual in English and French, and there was simultaneous interpretation of all verbal communications and translation of all documents.

Though it was a heavy programme, it was found that the majority of participants undertook all this and a great deal more, voluntarily, in small informal groups, and in personal consultations with members of the Faculty. The numerical level of attendance at sessions was good and members had enough energy left to take part in a few organized excursions and in private visits to the bathing beaches.

The work was divided into three phases. For the first week the emphasis of study was on normal child development patterns in France, the United Kingdom, and the United States, and a great deal of time was given to individual study of case material, with lectures devoted to supplementing the case material. For reasons of organization it became necessary to fit into this week sessions by Dr. René Spitz and Dr. Aubry (Dr. Roudinesco) on their work in connection with the separation of young babies from their mothers. This came as a shock to those members of the Seminar who were not familiar with this field. As things turned out, this unintended shock method was advantageous, in that it gave the Seminar an unforgettable experience of learning under stress. The balance was, to some extent, redressed by the lecturers who dealt with the normal living patterns of families in the three countries.

During the second week the emphasis shifted to a study of family phenomena, and in this phase the significant differences in cultural pattern became the centre of interest of the seminar. This aspect was specifically fostered by lectures and films on other cultural patterns up till then not described during the Seminar. In the third week the emphasis changed again towards a more practical aim, which was to consider those phenomena which underlie cultural change and how change may be brought about. Most of the participants in the Seminar had heavy responsibilities in the public health and child welfare administrations in their own countries, and in their professional work were continuously engaged in promoting measures designed to affect the life of their people, to change habits, and to improve conditions of life for children. These participants were familiar with the inadequacy of the traditional attitude that a proposed change is a good thing in its own right and that therefore people must adopt it, and they were anxious to discuss how to ensure that people will, in fact, adopt such a change. They had good reason to inquire what factors contribute towards, or detract from, the successful alteration of people's living habits.

These pressing questions were studied against the background of what happens when young babies are subjected to important circumstances of change, such as separation from their mothers,

7

and other studies were made in relation to the phenomena to be met with in children's groups. Knowledge derived from these fields was supplemented by studies of other cultures and particularly by studies of the impact of technological change on a primitive culture. Valuable lessons were learnt from these studies, about the process of social change and how it can be effected. The central thought of this part of the Seminar's work may be epitomized in an idea put forward by Dr. Margaret Mead, that Man, living in a changing environment, becomes a creature of change: now, for the first time in history, Mankind is self-conscious about social change, and Man is able to subject the details of his own behaviour to conscious scrutiny. Mental Health Services and other social services must be attuned to this period in which society is becoming aware of change, but it must be remembered how hard it is for people to give up their accustomed rhythms of living and to substitute self-consciousness for listening to the voice of tradition. The task of modern society is to make new inventions, to help build a new culture of change which will maintain the balance between the inside and the outside world.

THE WORKING GROUPS

The five working groups were as heterogeneous in composition as it was possible to make them, but much thought was given to their composition and to their working method. It is well-known, for example, that to get the best tangible results, the most cogent and effective report and the most sensible and progressive conclusions, a group needs to be homogeneous in culture, professional training and aim, but that such a group will add little to the general and cultural education of its members. On the other hand, where the group is too heterogeneous, group processes, i.e., those phenomena which arise out of the existence of the group and its engaging in a common task, may cause great difficulties in mutual understanding.

In the various preparatory discussions held in advance of the Seminar, it was agreed that the main aim was an educative one: to widen the horizon of the participants and to give them ideas for application in their own countries. It was not required that the groups should produce a formal report at the end of their period of work, though they were free to do so if they wished. It was also agreed that it was not sensible to set up very heterogeneous groups, and expect them to have a constructive and useful meeting, without some preparation.

Having decided that, with all their drawbacks, heterogeneous groups were best for the purposes of the Seminar, the solution adopted was a compromise, in that participants were given a period in which to settle down. The first groups were temporary, participants being placed in five ethnic groups and, when numbers made it possible, these were subdivided by profession. The purpose of this preliminary group meeting was to discuss the nature of group processes and to allow members of the Faculty an opportunity of meeting participants. The Faculty members were then able to choose the more permanent groups on a basis of heterogeneity of race, language and profession, but avoiding at the same time any obvious personality clashes.

Apart from the appointment of Group Chairmen from among the Faculty, and apart from their planned heterogeneity, there was little formal structure given to the groups, which were left to work out their own methods. This presented considerable difficulty to those participants—the majority—who had no previous experience of discussion groups even in their own countries, let alone in an international setting. Being left to work out their own method of procedure, they naturally varied a great deal. Groups were given thirteen working periods of about two hours, spread over the eighteen working days, and three reporting sessions were proposed, in which each group was to give a progress report to the full Seminar. In fact, the first of these reporting sessions, at the end of the first week, was by common consent, not used. These groups had an experience similar to that of most continuing discussion groups in such a setting. In the first week all the groups plunged into their task with great enthusiasm, wished for more time for group work, and were, perhaps, critical of the amount of time given to lectures. Much of the participants' free time during this week was devoted to the study of case material, and they could be seen in small gatherings, continuing their group work at all hours. During the second week there was an air of discouragement and frustration about the group work. Participants felt that they had neglected the case material; that they were not getting to grips with their subject; that it was just a matter of 'hot air', and so on. During the last week the great majority recovered their nerve and their enthusiasm for the group method; the way ahead appeared to be clearer to them and, although some were under a self-imposed pressure to complete their report in time, the morale of all was high at the close. There was, however, a minority in each group, which was never really appreciative of the discussion method and which would have preferred an entirely didactic method of teaching. This might be found to relate closely to University practice in the countries of these participants.

It has been common experience at the conferences of the World Federation for Mental Health, that heterogeneous, multi-professional, cross-cultural groups tend to show regularly a cycle of this

9

nature; first a period of enthusiasm, secondly a period of frustration and a negative attitude, and thirdly, miraculously appearing towards the close of the conference, a recovery of morale leading to a sense of satisfaction at the end. The length of time may vary between five and twenty days, but so long as it is known to the participants in advance, duration does not appear to make any difference to the periodicity of this phenomenon.

WORKING GROUP REPORTS

The five working groups produced, under pressure of time, statements which illustrated the different working methods which they had adopted, and their reports must be taken, not so much as evidence of what the groups did with the material, as of what they considered would interest the rest of the Seminar. Thus, these reports do not refer to the learning processes within the group, the amount of study of the case material, nor the technicalities under discussion.

Group A gave its report in the form of nineteen points on which they collectively thought that action could usefully be taken. These points, though perhaps not highly original in themselves, were all practical; and if they could be acted upon in each country with only a moderate degree of success, they would bring about a beneficent social revolution in the countries concerned. It was recognized, however, that action could only be taken by groups of people belonging to the countries.

Group B was concerned more with professional techniques and was self-conscious also about the actual process of communication within the group. They were concerned, for example, that in carrying out their work social workers must be prepared to listen rather than to give advice, and might be better employed carrying their services to the home rather than persuading the client to visit the office. The self-consciousness of the group about group dynamics can be illustrated by a quotation from the report: 'though, of course, we did not come to any remarkable conclusions, we felt that during the week we were able to discuss more easily.' Here is a practical example of the effectiveness of learning under stress.

This group considered the cultural pattern as a problem in itself and came to the conclusion that the participant in the Seminar who merely wanted proven facts to enrich his store of factual knowledge to take home with him, was missing the point of the Seminar. He was not recognizing that greater awareness of cultural phenomena which students of the behavioural sciences, and social welfare workers generally, must have. The effectiveness of the group method in enabling its members to come to conclusions which are full of insight can be illustrated by another quotation, this time from a report on a discussion about a certain type of institution for young children: 'It looks as if one is deliberately making delinquents.'

Group C reported on more general conclusions than the two foregoing, and was concerned with the relevance of mental hygiene to the current state of the world. This group postulated, for example, that a mental hygiene programme needs an 'under-structure' before it can be effective; in other words, child guidance clinics cannot be suitable for primitive communities where there are no other agencies to deal with cruder problems, and where the community has no concept of how to use clinics. Such a conclusion took this group on to the realization that its participants, like those referred to in group *B* above, also could not hope to take back to their own countries ready-made solutions for application on the spot, but that they could take back with them a fresh orientation to their work.

Group D reported in more practical terms, in relation to the actual work method which appeared most suitable for achieving the aims of its members. They decided that, in particular, the method of community centres was the most effective for the countries from which they themselves came. This led the group to advocate a rationalization of the social provisions of the community and the canalization of all social work through one single multi-purpose type of worker. This conclusion arose out of the group's sense of the ineffectiveness of purely curative methods, especially those of child guidance, when faced with living problems in the community. They also considered the mental hygiene problems of the worker himself but did not, apparently, consider those of the lone worker in a primitive community. The position of such a person in any community is unenviable.

Group E applied itself consciously to the techniques of conferences and considered cultural differences and ways to overcome them; it also attempted to evaluate the phenomena of warmth and friendliness as a means of estimating the value of conference procedure. It is interesting that this group felt the need to preface its report with a defensive explanation of why it had spent much of its time on this. It appeared likely that this was because of a division, within the group, on working method; a minority had wished for a precise and directed discussion, whereas the majority had wished for a free and permissive work method. The report which they produced arose out of the discussion to resolve this difficulty, and appeared to them, as indeed to all the other members of the Seminar, to represent an ever-present issue in international work. The group was in unanimous agreement about the usefulness and personal significance of the experience of together working through these differences of approach and opinion and arriving at a formulation of the problem, if not a final solution.

OTHER ADMINISTRATIVE ARRANGEMENTS

It was thought desirable that the control of the Seminar by the Director and Faculty be tempered by a consultative committee of five elected representatives of the participants and five Faculty members, to report to the Faculty and make suggestions, comments and criticisms. Nothing came out of this to affect the general structure of the programme but a number of alterations in detail were suggested and adopted, which enabled the participants to feel a more direct sense of control of the Seminar.

Throughout the three weeks' period a minimum of regulations was introduced. A number of participants expressed the wish to be allowed to read papers and to call special meetings to consider some specific subject. So far as was possible they were given facilities to do this on the understanding that attendance was purely voluntary. Two members read prepared papers to small groups of this sort, and a number of other informal meetings and discussions were held.

KENNETH SODDY,

Director of the Seminar.

Part Two

CHILD
DEVELOPMENT
PATTERNS

France

CHILD DEVELOPMENT PATTERNS IN FRANCE. (I)

Juliette Favez-Boutonier

THE TYPICAL French child does not exist. Children in France differ very much according to the region in which they were born; there are considerable cultural differences between the little villages far away in Brittany and those in the south or south-west of France, or, again, in the north. There is a great variety of regional environments and, of course, of social backgrounds. Standards of living vary according to the economic situation, education and knowledge vary, and all this goes to make up a complex regional background. I think it is impossible to give a complete or accurate idea of the general pattern of child development in France, so I must apologise in advance for what can only be partial and personal conclusions.

In these two commentaries I shall draw upon both groups of documents prepared for the Seminar, so as to point out certain factors which influence the way in which the child is reared and taught. In spite of the great variety to which I have referred, there is, nevertheless, a relative uniformity amongst French children; and even though we may say that a typical French child does not exist, yet there are subtle differences which make us feel that the French child is not quite the same as the English child or the Italian child. These differences become clearer as the child grows older, for up to the age of two years they are very slight. Our reason for choosing to study the very young child at the Seminar was the hope of tracing the causes of these differences to their source, of determining the influences that make the child develop along certain lines, that stamp him with the hallmark of a particular culture and make him an integrated member of the social group to which he belongs.

When we try to discover what influences affect the child during his early development, in France, we usually find that regional factors stand out—those, for instance, which distinguish the south of France from Brittany. However, regional characteristics of the sort I have in mind hardly appear at all in the material at our disposal, for these inquiries were mostly made in the neighbourhood

15

of Paris and the country near by; but from my own studies I have non-statistical material about regional factors to which I shall refer from time to time.

There are two other groups of factors to take into account: first, the social background, the various social classes determined by the parents' trade or profession, by their level of education and, generally speaking, by their culture; secondly, the family factors, depending on the structure of the family and the atmosphere created within it by the relations between the parents, and the way these affect the children.

One may wonder, when a child is born, how his mother proposes to bring him up, especially if she has not had a child before. Instinct, as we all know, plays no part in this matter. You do not have to teach a cat, a dog, or any other female animal, how to look after its young, although domestic animals, it is true, are not always very clever at bringing them up; but for women there is no ready-made solution.

Observation of how a mother sets about tackling the situation shows that there are three possibilities: first, she may say: 'I will do as my mother did', and she may copy her mother's methods or her grandmother's or those of some other older woman who brought her up. She feels that the right way to care for children is common knowledge, and she will do for her children the same as was done for her. So she adopts the habits, traditional methods and social code (usually fairly rigid) of the group in which she lives, confident that the group has had experience and that all she has to do is to follow its rules.

Secondly, she may feel that the way to bring up children is something that has to be learnt, and say to herself: 'I will ask the people who know—the paediatrician or the midwife.'

Thirdly, and this happens among people who are perhaps more aware of the educational problems involved, the mother may say to herself: 'This is a question that I must study. I know that bringing up a child is a very complicated business, and I will try to be really scientific about it.'

So there are generally these three groups of people, but my own experience shows that there is still another type, though it is more rare: they are the people who are fanatical about some particular system, for example, naturists or vegetarians, or those who take up this or that idea, sure that it will provide the solution of the problem of bringing up their children. The strangest example of this type that I have ever seen was a mother who brought up her child exclusively on almond milk.

The social study brings out these three main psychological attitudes, and deals with an educated circle of psychologist-parents, a working-class group in a town and a comfortably-off group in the country; but the middle class, the liberal professions, and the level of culture slightly lower than that of the well-off rural groups, are lacking. However, these missing groups also fall into my three main types. Among the very poor classes you may find a degree of submission to routine and tradition which amounts almost to resignation. The parents not only do what has always been done, but only what was actually done for themselves. They know roughly what is customarily done for children and they do not attempt anything else.

On the other hand, in well-to-do middle-class and professional circles, where women have jobs, or have a role to play in society, their days are full and they cannot look after their children all the time, so they employ a trained children's nurse. In the end the result is the same: either they will engage an old-fashioned nannie, or someone who has herself been brought up on lines of which they approve, or, if they are 'modern', somebody who is technically qualified.

Does the inquiry indicate that the parents' attitudes have any effect on the up-bringing of the children? Do they in practice have any great effect on the way in which these children are prepared for life and fitted for their cultural environment?

It seems that there is no significant variation in the clothing and feeding of the children: all French children wear swaddling clothes for a time, but these are soon left off in the daytime, though continued at night for a considerable time. As regards feeding, they are breast-fed at first but soon put on to a mixed diet; and in this the various social circles are about the same. With regard to material equipment, the influence of child welfare work has resulted in the use of play-pens, and of special children's chairs and spoons to about the same extent at all levels; the French peasant's child has toys similar to those of other children, provided that his parents can afford them.

Where can we find any really marked difference? There is of course the question of baths. Peasants' children do not usually have baths, but then neither do their parents. The children are washed but not bathed, and this is general among the rural population of France, and perhaps also in some urban working-class areas.

In towns the chamber pot is used, but it is quite unknown in some country districts. When the child is tiny he relieves himself wherever he happens to be, in the farmyard or indoors on the floor; and when he grows up he uses the same utensils as his parents. They do not usually buy him anything special, because this seems to them superfluous.

C   17

In the country also they do not bother with apparatus to help the child to stand: children play in the farmyard and have not very far to fall. They are less exposed to the danger of accidents than town children, and can crawl about on the grass, so the parents do not think it necessary to guard against their falling.

One notices the absence of the dummy in urban areas, but in the country its use seems to persist. In spite of the legal prohibition of the use of dummies, in France, peasants always manage to give their children one. The reasons appear to be practical—it probably stops the children from crying and makes them less troublesome.

Other articles whose use is unknown in the country, are waterproof knickers, politely called 'a protective device' in the report. Protective devices are used in all circles at night to keep the baby from wetting the bed, but waterproof knickers are not used by day in country districts. The child normally roams around without any 'protective device' at all, in fact without any knickers, to save washing. This solution of the problem is peculiar to country districts, and though it may happen in some working-class districts, it is probably less usual there because there is not so much room for the child to run about in. In the country a child without knickers does not create any problems of dirt—in fact it makes less work for the mother.

And now, how does the child develop? We find that in these conditions, which do not differ very much from each other, development, in some respects, is identical. For instance, the average development quotient is the same in all three groups—viz. 100—in spite of differences in the parents' cultural level and education. Similarly, the average age at which the child can walk is exactly the same in all three groups, i.e., 13 months. M. Zazzo draws certain conclusions from this: he observes that when children are learning to walk they are taught in different ways according to the circumstances in which they live. In the town they have little supports on wheels (*baby trotts*) or play-pens, and there is a tendency to teach them to walk young; but this does not make any difference in the way the faculty of walking develops, or in the age by which the child can walk by itself. The proportion of children who crawl before walking is exactly the same, and the average age at which they walk is 13 months, in all three groups. M. Zazzo concludes that the ability to walk results from an inward process of development on which cultural influences have a minimal effect. This conclusion is supported by ethnological studies of the average age at which children learn to walk in very different cultural environments, in some of which they have much less opportunity than in others, to move about before they reach the walking stage.

Dr. Jackson seems to take a slightly different view, as she thinks that now-a-days in the United States there is a tendency to try to hasten this particular form of development, and to make children walk earlier. This is a point for discussion, and I think it ought to be stressed that in France neither parents nor paediatricians try to get children to walk earlier. I would even go so far as to say that parents are inclined to think that as long as the child cannot walk, things are more likely to be peaceful and quiet. Of course, they are pleased when the child does walk, but one month earlier or later does not worry them, and they feel, on the contrary, that as long as the child cannot get around there is less risk of damage than there will be later when he starts to walk. There is even a feeling amongst paediatricians, though it is not common, that early walking is bad for the child and may make him develop bow legs. This belief is fairly widespread amongst the French public. Obviously the happy medium needs to be found between the tendency to make children walk early, and to prevent them from walking when they are capable of it. In France at present we think it is quite reasonable for children to walk at about one year old, and that there is no need to encourage them to do so sooner.

When we come to the subject of toilet-training, we find differences. Toilet-training begins earlier in the urban working-class and in the better educated group than it does in the country. Children acquire clean habits much earlier in the working-class family, or at any rate in the type of family dealt with in this study; and the conclusion is drawn that the three groups reach this stage at different ages. Children in rural areas begin to be trained relatively late, whereas town parents begin the training in the child's first months. Half the country parents scarcely trouble about it at all, and the country children, living uncramped lives in close proximity to domestic animals, gain control later than those in the town. For the town dwellers, toilet-training seems to cause more trouble than any other process and causes the greatest number of scenes between parents and children. It is the form of discipline most highly rated in urban environments and least sought after in the country. In the latter, cleanliness at night is of some account, but not so much in the daytime. In the living-rooms of French farms, where from time to time the chickens come in and deposit their little offerings, never mind where, the fact that the child does the same is not likely to bother anybody. You wash or sweep up once a day—it is quite simple. At night, making a mess gives more trouble; even so no one really bothers about it.

The figures given in the report are what might be expected; some children are toilet-trained from 6 months onwards, but you can

19

train children even earlier. In the east of France, and in particular in Alsace, where the people perhaps are more keen on discipline and cleanliness, the results achieved are sometimes amazing. In one case in which a child had been toilet-trained by the age of 3 weeks, the mother had observed very closely at what moments the gastro-colic reflex occurred and had noticed that the child tended to evacuate as soon as he had had his bottle, perhaps even while taking his bottle. She therefore placed him on the pot at the same time as giving him the bottle, and in this way she created a conditioned reflex: when put on the pot, the child evacuated. She was very pleased with the results until, when the child was about one year old, the family went to stay with the grandmother and forgot the precious pot. The child then firmly refused to oblige. He was trained to his little pot and to nothing else. This was a catastrophe, for nothing happened for twenty-four hours and they had to go home and fetch the pot. Then later, at the age of 13, that boy became very passive, was not doing well at school, and was in general getting on very badly. Though he had developed normally until 2 or 3 years old, later on, in spite of being more than averagely intelligent, he developed this passive attitude and seemed to have no personal initiative. I do not know whether there was any connection between these things, but to my mind there seemed to be a problem there.

Is the fact that it is possible for a child to be trained at a very early age a valid reason for wishing every child to have clean habits at the age of 3 weeks or a month? Do we think that very early train-ing is helpful to personality development? My own views are not unbiassed: I have seen so many disturbed children who had under-gone this exceptionally early training that I think it is essential that research should be done to find out whether there are any advantages in striving for clean habits before the normal age. Personally I suspect that there are disadvantages. For indeed if toilet-training is to be an educational process and not a mere training, it must be carried out in conditions other than the simple acquisition of a conditioned reflex. For example, this child who was trained at the age of 3 weeks and refused to use anything except his own little pot at the age of 1 year, had certainly been placed at a disadvantage in relation to other children—the disadvantage of the limiting of his behaviour, with no psychological enrichment, and no freedom of choice. Training, even by insidious means, imposes a certain type of fixed behaviour, while education offers, and stimulates in the child, appropriate and flexible modes of behaviour, which he can select rather than obey blindly.

Toilet-training is a phase in a child's life in which he chooses to become clean, and it can only be an educational experience when he is consciously doing something that he understands. Even if he is reprimanded when he is dirty, it is still an appeal to his personal capacity to choose between one thing and another; but if he becomes a little automaton who evacuates the moment he is put on a pot, I do not see where any education comes in. It amounts to no more than stimulating a physiological and psychological activity for which the child's personality is not yet ready. I put this idea forward with certain reservations. Toilet-training is one of the points which vary most in France, according to social environment, region, and parents, and research into this matter would be very interesting.

We now come to sleep. In France the child usually sleeps in his parents' room when he is very small, mainly of necessity on account of insufficient accommodation, even in the country. Country dwellings do not have many rooms. There is plenty of space on the farm for barns, stables and outhouses, but there is very little accommodation for the people themselves, so the baby often sleeps in his parents' room. (This is not mentioned in our study, but is my personal experience.) The time at which the child is put to bed varies; some parents are very strict, some put their children to bed at the same time winter and summer, some change the hour in accordance with the season—particularly in the country, where the daylight is important—and some children have a rest in the afternoon during their second year while others do not. The afternoon rest has some relationship with the crying and screaming by night and day, which is mentioned in the report. Generally speaking, young children rest or sleep in the afternoon for quite a long time, although always less regularly in the country than in the town. The need for a little quiet makes the mother put the child to bed, even if it does not want to sleep.

The inquiry into feeding habits brings out the important point that weaning takes place later in the country than in the town. There is less regularity about feeding, and a bottle may be given even after the age of one year. Thus, those who follow traditional methods most closely are less rigid about weaning, while those who try to be up-to-date, and follow scientific or pseudo-scientific developments or instructions are more strict about stopping the bottle. In my experience many children in different environments are still weaned very late, and are given a bottle for quite a long time after they have been weaned. Sometimes this becomes quite pathological: recently I saw a boy—not a country boy—who insisted upon having his bottle every day until he was 10. Nevertheless he is neither abnormal nor backward, although not particularly well adjusted. Up to the age of 4 or 5, in fact until school age, it is quite common to find a child wanting a bottle. Very little attention is paid to this, especially

21

in the country. One might ask whether paediatricians and modern child welfare clinics, in encouraging the parent to get the child to give up sucking as soon as possible, and to use a spoon or a cup, to wean the child early and to vary the diet, take sufficient account of the child's need to suck, and to suck for quite a long time.

I think that the bottle itself and the circumstances in which it is given have not been sufficiently studied. Experiments have been made with puppies fed with bottles with different kinds of teats. Some of them had to make an effort and suck very hard because the holes were small, and others were given teats with big holes so that the milk came easily. The puppies who had to suck hardest developed the best, on the same quantity of milk, showing that the need to suck is related to needs which should be respected.

A fairly high proportion of French children who are weaned early, suck their thumbs or their fingers, or anything they can find. The inquiry shows that the proportion of children who suck their thumbs is fairly high, and M. Zazzo writes: 'If some of the parents attach most importance to the child's clean habits, some paediatricians and psychologists attach perhaps even greater importance to finger-sucking. According to the psychoanalysts, the pleasure derived from sucking apparently carries the child back as it were, to a Golden Age of infancy, while at the same time giving him, during his first year of life, useful experience of the possibilities for pleasure afforded by his mouth, since this sensory satisfaction would appear to constitute a normal stage in his psychological development. While almost all paediatricians agree in proscribing dummies, in the name of hygiene, most psychologists say that finger-sucking, which is normally given up between 2 and 3 years of age, should be allowed.' I do not agree that psychologists think it is a good thing for children to suck their thumbs. The report continues: 'Harsh intervention, through teasing or covering up the fingers, or punishment, may sow the first seed of neurosis in the child's psychological life.' I differ somewhat from this view: it is true that psychologists tell parents not to stop children sucking their fingers because the fact that they do it shows that they have a need for it. To try to stop finger-sucking is to risk harming the children rather than curing them; but it is still a problem for the psychoanalysts, to discover why children *need* to suck their fingers. The child who sucks his thumb must be unsatisfied in some way or other. Perhaps it is a return to the way in which he was fed in early infancy, or perhaps something induced by bottle-feeding rather than by breast-feeding. Our report ends by saying: 'We found that only half the children still sucked their fingers (preferably the thumb) between 1 and 2 years of age; that in seven of the twenty-eight cases noted, the parents tried to prevent it; that children who sucked their fingers were to be found in the "better educated" group rather more often than in either of the others, and that out of thirty-four children weaned before the age of 3 months, there were eighteen who sucked their fingers during their second year, or 53 per cent. Of twenty-six children weaned at 4 months, there were ten who sucked their fingers, or 38 per cent.' These statistics, although inadequate, suggest that the child tends to suck its fingers if it is weaned too early. I should like research to be done on this whole question, in other countries as well as in France.

To conclude, I will say something about obsessional behaviour traits, which are becoming more and more widespread in France. These are persistent personal habits: it may be that the child refuses to be separated from some object, or insists on certain fixed ways of doing things. It may sometimes be a special rite before going to sleep or having a bath (more usually the former). It may perhaps occur less frequently among country children, probably because they have more freedom, more opportunity to play with each other, and their life is less strictly controlled. Possibly this ritualism, as it might be termed, is really a response to that of the parents: in other words, parents who follow fixed rules for living which they impose on the children, may perhaps themselves provide the reason why the children develop this sense of ritual, though it may become very tiresome for them.

Obsessional habits are so common and so widespread that they cannot be regarded as pathological. Admittedly they do not exactly constitute an illness; but can we feel that they are desirable? Are they in a sense parasitic, like a flea, for example, which does not usually cause an illness, but which we would rather get rid of than keep? In fact, the child invents its ritual and clings to it even if it seems bad to us. We should try to get rid of these habits, but judiciously and without forcing the child to give up, suddenly, things of which, for the time being, he has a need. We do not know what sort of need the child is trying to satisfy by his ritual.

One further word, on punishments. In France I think smacking is fairly general. It is not very severe and is thought to be the simplest way of dealing with children. Punishments such as deprivation of food are not much favoured, especially since the war. It was so difficult to feed children then, that a feeling has remained that one should not deprive them of food. Putting them in a corner and telling them that nobody loves them is also done, but is not so general. The inquiry showed that even the highly educated parents, who reckon to bring up their children on principles, admitted, rather shamefacedly, that they occasionally smacked their children. Nevertheless, these parents preferred punishments of an affective, or moral, kind; but as the inquiry showed that their children were as difficult as those in other groups, we cannot draw any conclusions on the educational influence of punishments. The parents' characters certainly have as much influence as the type of punishment. Careful research would be necessary to determine this, but would be difficult to carry out. All these facts go to show to what extent the personal behaviour of the parents has to be considered as well as more strictly social factors, in order to understand the development of the child's personality.

CHILD DEVELOPMENT PATTERNS IN FRANCE. (II)

Juliette Favez-Boutonier

MY PREVIOUS PAPER led us to the conclusion that the patterns of development of the child are not fixed, whatever the social background may be; and that the family background cannot be separated from the social background. Whatever the importance of the social background for the child, and especially for the child of less than 2 years of age, the family background acts as a kind of filter which allows only certain things to reach the child. As such, it might be likened to the mother's placenta, an organ which ensures that the child receives what it needs, even to the detriment of the mother, since the child may be better fed than the mother. The result may be that even in fairly modest family backgrounds the children are very 'spoilt', surrounded with very great care and attention, because the parents make many sacrifices so that the children may not go through what they themselves endured. This family 'filtration' is easy up to the age of 2 years but after that it becomes more difficult because the child begins to move outside the family, and has progressively more direct contact with outside influences.

We have seen that the conditions of life and the living quarters are very important, that is to say, the influences, subject to variations, that depend upon the behaviour of the parents. The absence of playing space, for instance, may be compensated for by the attitude of the mother. Her tolerance, or severity with the child, is more important than the amount of space the child has to play in. On the other hand, the behaviour of the parents creates a sort of small universe, limited to the family itself, which will influence the child continuously, and in a very direct manner. So we may say that family life can be relatively independent of the conditions of social life, provided that the material and economic circumstances of the family are above a certain minimal level.

Of the cases described by Dr. Aubry[1] and her colleagues, I will now single out for consideration Danielle, who is 17 months old, and Alain, 15 months, both of whom come from an urban working-class background. It is obvious that the space in which children can move around is much larger in a rural environment than among

[1] See Vol. II, Part II.

city workers. Moreover, in a working-class family the parents are more severe in some respects, they stop the children doing some of the things that they want to do, as for instance in the matter of clean habits. One might think, therefore, that a child who lives in the country would always have a better motor development and a much freer attitude in general, than the child in the working-class background. During the survey the things forbidden to children were counted: on the average there were twenty-nine things forbidden among industrial workers, twenty-seven among the intellectuals, and seventeen among the rural workers. So the less space there was, the more things were forbidden, which, one might think, would lead to greater inhibitions and slower development of walking. But in the two cases mentioned, the impression is quite different: Danielle has a Locomotion Quotient of 99. She lives in an urban working-class environment, with very little space, but, in the view of the psychologist who tested her, the character of the mother, a rather anxious person, probably had some bearing on her retardation. Alain, however, lives in even worse material conditions than Danielle. Father, mother, the boy and a baby girl, live in one room (plus a very small kitchenette) on the ground floor of a big building. The room measures 3 metres by 2 metres 50 (10 ft. by 8 ft. 6 in.): the toilets, used in common with other tenants, are in the passage outside. The room does not even have normal daylight but requires electric light all day; there is no garden; and life for the three people, with a 2-months' old baby, who live in it, must be exceedingly difficult. In spite of this, Alain has a Locomotion Quotient of 105. He appears, therefore, to be developing more rapidly than Danielle. It might be expected that these two children in such a small dwelling space, and living in the suburbs, would be very sociable; but Danielle is only moderately sociable whereas Alain is confident and open-natured. It seems again, that the mother's attitude must play an important part in this, for she is very healthy, young, competent and active.

Now let us look at two cases from a rural background. First of all another Alain[1] who is 14 months old and lives under quite good material conditions with his mother and father, twin sisters aged $8\frac{1}{2}$ years, and a brother aged 4 years, in a large four-roomed house with a yard, and some land. The mother is an anxious person, whose own home life as a child was disturbed, and who is resentful of the family's present style of living, which is rather isolated, with few friends. Alain's Locomotion Quotient is merely the average one of 101, and he is inhibited and shy with strangers. Can this inhibition, this fear of strangers, be due to his life in the country, lack of contact

---

[1] A case-history studied at the Seminar, but not included in Vol. II.

with other people and little opportunity to meet new situations? No, for if the case of Yves[1], 15 months old, is compared, it will be seen that he is also of a rural background but his Locomotion Quotient is 128, as might be expected of a child brought up in the country, even if his material conditions are not outstandingly good. This family has only two rooms, with a large kitchen and a yard. The mother is active and lively, highly strung and excessively emotional; but she is very affectionate towards the children, possessive rather than dominating, and a slave to them. Yves runs in and out, and his attitude towards strangers is smiling and confident. It is reasonable to surmise that this is influenced by the family atmosphere.

A certain correlation now becomes apparent between the behaviour of the parents and the kind of development of the child. I say the 'kind of development' because these children are neither seriously backward nor retarded. In all the case-histories there has been only Case No. 1[2], where the child weighed too little at birth and was poorly developed, perhaps mainly on account of organic factors. In the other eight or nine cases of fairly normal development, it is evident that there is a relationship between the behaviour of the child while being tested, and the attitude of the mother and father towards the child, and to a lesser degree the attitudes of brothers and sisters. Let us say that the personality of the child is deeply influenced by the nature of his relationship with his family, and particularly with his mother and father.

Now let us consider the effect of this maternal attitude, which I would prefer to call the maternal function, because it is more an influence of whoever takes the part of the mother than a personal influence. In a good number of cases, the grandparents reinforce, complement or correct the attitude of the mother in looking after the children, when they are living with the family. This situation is not so common in towns because of lack of room, but there are very many working-class and middle-class families in France in which the children are brought up in part or wholly by the grandparents. For example, in one of our families the child spends a great part of its time with the grandparents, who are neighbours, so two adult feminine influences are working on him. However, this situation is not limited to rural families: in many urban working-class families a grandmother plays a very important part in the upbringing of the child. Dr. Margaret Mead has said that it is important to know whether the children are, in fact, brought up by the parents, the grandparents, brothers or sisters. In France, far more than statistics show, children who are not completely orphans are brought up by

---

[1] See Vol. II, Part II.
[2] A case-history studied at the Seminar, but not included in Vol. II.

the grandparents. This may be because the mother is not living, but, more often, because she is working and gives her child, while very young, to her parents to be brought up in the country. Many city-born children are shown in the statistics, at the age of 4 or 5, as urban children, but up to that age they have been brought up by the grandparents in the country. In the past the grandparents were able to come to live in the cities and bring the children up there, but now material circumstances are less favourable.

Very often an elder sister plays the part of the mother to a great extent, and having feminine reactions and feminine psychology she plays a protecting and educating role in the child's life. I do not know what 'feminine' really means, but in our society it is more often the daughter who imitates the mother and adopts the maternal attitude than the son; and so it is a phenomenon of imitation which one must take into account. The maternal personality seems to have echoes in other persons in the family, and all these together constitute the maternal element in the life of the child, which will form its character. One of the children whom we studied had a sister of 5 who looked after him a lot as soon as he was no longer a baby in arms. The attitude of this 5-year-old sister appeared to be very favourable; she was able to compensate for what was, perhaps, some over-anxiousness in the mother.

In addition to the maternal there is the paternal function. This takes second place, though not necessarily so after the age of 2. Of course, the mother looks after the child most of the time but the complementary influence of the father is certainly as necessary as that of the mother. In our case-histories, the influence of the father can often be seen completing, correcting, and balancing the influence of a nervous or anxious mother. This aspect of the father's attitude has a direct influence on the child, but can be served also by a grandfather or an older brother, though there is not actually an example of the latter in our case-histories. It can be said that the paternal influence is independent of the father-mother relationship; that is, that the father acts as an educator in himself. But to emphasize this would be to miss the main point: the father is not only a man who lives close to the child, he is the husband of the mother, and that is the essential element of the family structure. What is the nature of this combination? Husband and wife living together are not only two people engaged in bringing up the child, they are bound to each other by ties which must counterbalance, so to speak, those which exist between the mother and the child and between the father and the child, but particularly the former. This two-sided education is successful only if each brings up the child, not in order to keep the child for herself or himself, as a sort of personal property, but in order to 'give' the child to the other. This way of putting it goes beyond my meaning, perhaps, but I wish to imply that the person who brings up the child must give the impression that she is not going to cling to it, but will let it go ahead into its own future. The best way of doing this is to be able to give the child to the father, and the same principle applies to the father also. This attitude of mutual gift is only possible if there is a real partnership, where husband and wife are satisfied with each other and reveal in their attitude towards the child this feeling of a reciprocal gift. The mother, in the care of the child, not only does not become detached from the father but is doing something for him: and the father, when he plays with or helps the child, is also doing something for the mother. This is the parental aspect of what has been called the Oedipus complex, in which the parents play their part as well as the children. There are parents, especially mothers, who cling to their children and who think that the child is essentially their property, particularly if they do not get on well with their husbands. This is the parental Oedipus complex which does not allow the child to emancipate itself from the mother.

I will not enlarge on this subject, but let us try and see what has happened in the cases I have quoted, and how the attitude of the parents and their mutual relationship have influenced the children. Danielle, who is an inhibited child, is the daughter of a couple whose married life has never been satisfactory. The mother married without love. She had been in love with a man whom she felt she was going to marry, but he was unfaithful, and married another woman. Danielle's mother continued to love this man, though without thought of being unfaithful to her husband. She had had considerable difficulties already in her own family: her father was an alcoholic, who continually quarrelled with her mother, whom she idealised. The man whom she married also had difficulties. When he was 9 his mother died in his presence, but the father was not there, being out with another woman whom he subsequently married. The son never forgave his father for having been unfaithful to her, so he too, in a way, has a fixation, on his mother. He gets on so badly with his wife that divorce is being considered.

Danielle would be even more deeply scarred by this unfortunate family situation if she did not have a sister a little older than herself. This child does not seem to be well balanced, but has, perhaps, found in her younger sister a means of expressing herself a little, by identifying herself with the mother and becoming a better mother than the real one, while Danielle finds a mother substitute in the older sister.

Now let us examine the case of Alain, of whom I said that his development was much more satisfactory than the material conditions could have led one to hope. Alain is a happy child, in good health, contented, like everyone else in that home. The parents get on together very well; they are young and in love with each other; there is evidence of this in the fact that the child was conceived before marriage. This, in the present day life of young people in France, of this social class, is no proof of immorality. Homes are difficult to find and very often these couples, who, under more normal circumstances would have married, are led into situations of this kind because of bad social conditions. When the marriage is hurried by pregnancy, relations between their own parents and the young couple are sometimes strained, but in this case it seems that the former made it easy for the couple to marry. They lived at first with one of the older families until this little apartment was found. The husband works hard, is sober, and enjoys sport and company. The wife is young, active, and very lively; she manages to make quite a home out of this one miserable room, balances her budget and gives small presents to her family without particularly counting the cost. She is always dressed in good taste, looks attractive, and enjoys life.

On looking into the family life of these two young people, it appears that the mother has always had a very happy relationship with her own mother. Her parents have been a happily married couple. The husband's parents also got on well and he is fond of them—not over-devoted, but his relationship with them is good. The grandparents on both sides help the young couple whenever they can, but do not interfere in their affairs. We can see from these two cases how behaviour of the parents has a strong influence on the children, but how this behaviour has already been influenced by their own childhood background: an influence which acts in a 'longitudinal' dimension, so to speak, over the years, in contrast with statistics which make a sort of 'transverse section' in time and take note of things at a given moment.

Should most importance be attached, then, to social factors or to family factors? The cases we have examined seem to show that, up to the age of 2, the family background, or atmosphere and style of life, are of greater importance for the child's development than the social background, but only when there is at least a minimum level of material security. It would not be true in cases of destitution, under-nutrition, or if the parents were mentally defective; and I must add that I would never say that no matter how poor the living accommodation, all will go well if the parents live in good humour! Because Alain's mother manages to make a home out of a tiny room, I would not advise the French Government to make all families with young parents live like that. Of course, people must have decent houses, but it will be found that even in good material conditions there can be mothers whose influence will have bad effects on their children's development.

Mme. Aubry suggests that the normal development of a child is brought about to a great extent by the family background. The term 'normal development' has little real meaning in psychology. All these children except one are of normal development and yet they are all different: there are subtleties of personality development which tests do not reveal. With the same development quotient, some children may give a good impression, seem happy and well adapted to life, while others appear much less well prepared for life. I do not yet know how we can try to examine these complex factors of personality development in greater detail. The complete examination of children—psychological, sociometric, etc.—is complicated and takes a very long time.

I would add that we have no means of evaluating the family development pattern: the results of social inquiries must be accepted with reserve, because the social workers, though conscientious, may be mistaken if they have not been properly trained in observation. They may see the home of a couple who do not fight, who are not overheard quarrelling and whose home is clean, so they note this down as a good home. I once saw, in prison, a young criminal who, at the age of 15 had murdered an old woman. The social workers, at the time he was condemned, reported that he had good parents, who were happy together, and had brought up their child well. When the young man was transferred to another prison eleven or twelve years later, another social worker visited the parents and found neighbours ready to talk. She found out that the mother was a paranoiac and got on badly with the father. It was a very carefully kept home, obsessionally clean, but the home life of this boy had been absolutely infernal, with a mother who had had a disastrous influence over him. Gross errors can clearly be made if the inquiry does not reveal the structure of the family in depth. This cannot be done purely by statistics and by observations of the material conditions of life of the family.

At the statistical level, we must take the results of the inquiry with reserve for two reasons. In the first place the background called rural is not really rural, but consists of agricultural workers who live not very far from a big metropolis. Country people living close to a city like Paris are not real peasants: they have no body of local traditions like other regions farther from the capital. These people tend to retain the faults of peasants rather than their good qualities. The industrial workers, on the other hand, give a very pleasant impression, but one wonders whether a comparable inquiry in a big industrial centre in the north or east of France would give similar results. Moreover, half of the women and men studied are the children of farming people, and this is the first generation with a workers' background, one in which the parents are still marked by the culture pattern of their rural background.

The observers remark on the great emotional warmth of these workers towards their children. Of all the families studied, the children of the working people seem to be most loved, and these fathers, in spite of the very little time spent at home, play most with their children. I wonder if this is not a reflection of an attitude that is deeply French, part of the tradition of the country people and the craftsmen, but which lies outside modern industrial life. These parents do things for their children out of a strong feeling, a pattern of behaviour originating in an age-old tradition still existing in France, that of giving oneself up to one's child. In some of the working-class families it is reported that the mother devoted herself entirely to the child: and though this attitude would not be true of all workers, it corresponds to a way of life characteristic of French people, of which one tends to find less, but which has left traces, and has perhaps resulted in there being, in France, so many families with only one child. Parents give themselves so much trouble over this child and make so many sacrifices, that one child is enough. It is thought quite normal for a mother to sacrifice herself to the child completely and give up all her time to it, and the father also; but he does it in his own way, without taking part in the management of the home. The inquiry shows that it is typical for a working-class father to spend a lot of time with the child and to play with it a great deal, but not to help the mother in looking after it. He will help her in other things but not in that; that is not his role.

On the other hand, among the families of higher education, less influenced by tradition and more progressive, the appearance of a new type of behaviour and of upbringing can be seen. There is a break with tradition and a search for something different and more rational. These parents attach great importance to the child but in a different manner; they do things for the child out of a sense of duty rather than pleasure, a feeling that such things should be done in a certain way, almost scientifically. The mother plays less with the children and gives less time to them. The father, who according to the inquiry probably has more time at home than the working-class father, plays less with the children but takes a greater share in looking after them. He is able to change the child's diapers, feed it, and so on, which indicates that the relationship of the couple is different. Hence there are two different types of family structure, both in need of further study. For example, it is the working-class parents who embrace their children the most, both the father and the mother, according to the inquiry. But we do not know whether the same loving relationship is true of the parents between themselves also. Both patterns have advantages and disadvantages. Probably for the very young child the traditional emotional attitude has most advantages, but I am not sure that this would be true after the age of 2. Moreover, in both cases the attitude of the parents towards the child remains controlled by something difficult to define—a kind of identification with it. In the one case the parents identify themselves with the child and tend to do what they think will please the child, and in the other case the more rationally behaved parents identify the child with themselves and tend to do what they think ought to be done for 'a little man'. But the former are doing at the same time something which pleases themselves, and the latter something that they think good from their own point of view. This goes to show that in order to help the parents with the upbringing and development of their children, one must strive to become independent of one's own emotional attitudes, which are able to make themselves felt though one's reasoning otherwise appears logical.

COMPARATIVE STUDY OF FRENCH CASE-HISTORIES

Jenny Aubry

IT IS IMPOSSIBLE to describe 'the American child', 'the English child', or the 'French child', because the 'typical' child does not exist. In Great Britain, and even more so in the U.S.A., which are geographically separated from the countries from which their immigrants come, the foreign elements bring with them many different customs and cultures, and their integration into the community sometimes gives rise to difficult problems. In France, on the other hand, there has been continual interchange with the neighbouring countries, and the cultural differences are less marked.

Habits and methods of rearing children in the north and east of France are undoubtedly affected by Germanic cultural practices, whereas in the south-east, immigrants are for the most part Italians, and in the south-west, Spaniards. The differences of custom between the north and the south of France are therefore very considerable, and are linked up with many, and very ancient, influxes of population.

The Parisian region, which we chose for study as a matter of convenience, also has its own peculiar characteristics. On the one hand, the highly centralized political and economic structure of France makes Paris a centre of attraction for people in the provinces, while at the same time, as a cultural and intellectual centre, it draws foreigners from every other country in the world. There are for example many foreign names in French literary, artistic and learned circles; but although the population is very mixed, it seems to fuse together in the melting-pot of the 'Ile de France', and produce a characteristically French culture.

Things are different among the working people, who, with the exception of certain types of skilled craftsmen, are less settled, and are for the most part employed in the lower grades of work, as labourers and seasonal agricultural workers or unskilled hands in industry.

In order to give a general idea of French cultural practices, we therefore chose at least partially skilled workmen in the urban setting, and agricultural labourers or country people living permanently in the district we had selected.

The town and country zones were chosen for the reason that most of the workmen of the Paris region are of recent peasant origin, in fact, removed from it by only one or two generations. Our task was to study the differences and similarities between these two settings and see whether we could find out how the changes and adjustments that are needed to settle in a new environment, were made.

Role of the Parents

In this respect the differences between the town and country families are not great. In both environments the mother plays the most important part in the home. She is mistress of the house, in charge of its upkeep and cleaning, responsible for the daily expenses and, in particular, for those connected with the family's food. In most cases the upbringing of the children during their first years, falls to her, and the rhythm and habits of the child's eating, sleeping, physical care, toilet-training and first education as a member of society, are regulated by her.

In the second year the mother generally has to deal with discipline, whereas later on she will rely on the father's authority. Nevertheless, if the mother reigns at home, it is the father who takes the lead in the family's social life. His opinion prevails whenever large expenditure is involved or decisions have to be taken about the way of living. It is he who takes part in trade union or political activities, and who meets his fellow-workers at the café in order to discuss work and politics.

Our ways are patriarchal; the father's name is handed down in our families, and the woman changes her identity when she marries. The civil code demands that the husband should succour and protect the wife, but she must give him obedience and faithfulness. Except under special contract, the family possessions in cash and kind are controlled by the husband, and in spite of recent modifications of the law, the same spirit pervades it still. But like the Roman matron, the French woman is respected in her home, and in it enjoys the prestige and authority invested in her by the head of the family.

Attitudes of the Mothers

The small number of cases studied makes it possible to draw only general assumptions from them, but these seem to be confirmed by the wider, though less detailed, studies of M. Zazzo and Professor Chombart de Lauwe,[1] and by the experiences of Mme. Favez-Boutonier.

It seems that two sets of conditions influence child-rearing practices:

[1] Part of the material used at the Seminar.

35

1. *Material and economic factors.* Living conditions in the country, even if they lack comfort, allow the child great freedom. In the sphere of motor development, he can move about without constraint, and with regard to cleanliness, country people are more tolerant than townspeople.

The fact, also, that in the country the woman is nearly always in her home, and her knowledge of the ways of animals, probably explain why feeding schedules are less rigid than in the town, and breast-feeding more common.

Country babies and town babies alike, are wrapped in swaddling clothes, but these are given up sooner in the town, probably under the influence of child-welfare teaching.

In France people like to eat well, and in town as well as country, more than three-fifths of their money is spent on food by wage earners. Lodging and clothes are of less importance. Except in the first few months of life, the diet is different from that in Anglo-Saxon countries; it comprises less milk and farinaceous foods and more animal protein. The need to prepare meals quickly, in present-day life in towns, has changed feeding habits to a certain extent.

Alcoholism is still a serious problem in France. From early childhood, children are given a little wine in their water, and in some provinces alcohol is even added to the feeding bottle. In spite of these habits, excessive drinking of spirits or alcohol is found, as in other countries, among people with personality problems.

2. *Parents' personality and its influence on the rearing and development of children.* One is struck, on reading the case-histories and the studies of the environments, by the small number of real differences between the rearing practices in one social class and another, and between those in the country and those in the town. Yet in spite of this, from the age of eighteen months, there are distinct differences in the behaviour of the children, and particularly in their relations with their parents. Another factor seems to come in; not so much what one does, or has done, for the child, as the way in which the mother puts her principles into practice.

For example, most mothers undertake toilet-training long before the child can understand what is wanted, well before the myelinisation of his nervous system is sufficiently advanced to allow of voluntary control of the sphincter muscles. In some cases this seems to have practically no ill effects on the child's character; in others, on the contrary, it gives rise to strong resistance, anger and enuresis. But these symptoms nearly always depend upon the degree of importance that the mother attaches to the success of her efforts. Some mothers put the child on the pot at three months old, but are not annoyed if this has no effect, and do not insist. Others, however, are determined to succeed, and try again and again, getting angry if the child does not respond in the way they want. These differences in attitude are not entirely rational, but in most cases depend upon the mothers' own relations in childhood with their parents, their conflicts and the way in which these were resolved. The case of Alain[1] is particularly interesting and enlightening in this respect.

There are similar examples in the notes on rigid feeding schedules, freedom to choose food, to move about and so on. They all derive from the same principle: some parents feel a compulsion to force certain habits on the child, not because they want to educate the child and make of him an independent individual, capable of adapting himself to the realities of life, but to satisfy their own needs.

Mme. Favez-Boutonier has emphasized the difference between educating and conditioning: I should like to stress that the urge to 'condition' a child often results from a badly resolved conflict between its parents and grandparents.

Besides this, changes of habit arising from a move from a country to a town way of living, make adjustments necessary. The studies show that parents who themselves had a happy childhood in harmonious family surroundings, which allowed for their development as mature persons, are the most capable of adapting to their new circumstances, without undue anxiety, the principles on which they were brought up.

On the whole we can say that in France, where conditions of life, in spite of industrialization, change less quickly than in the U.S.A., this adjustment seems to be accomplished without undue trouble; though it must be remembered that the losses incurred in two world wars, and the long absence from home of many of the fathers, have certainly changed in many ways the traditional structure of the family, and created problems that are sometimes very difficult to solve.

DISCUSSION

Material and economic factors: living conditions. In Lorraine, miners are housed by the mining companies, and have no choice but to remain; and, in the rural areas, proprietors and peasants remain on the soil. In Moselle, much damaged during the war, there are many different races in the industrial regions; Polish miners have retained their separate identity, and there is a small Polish school and cultural centre. There are migrants from Africa, Italians who have assimilated French culture, Russians and others. In one mining region, there had been an increase in the mortality of babies amongst displaced persons, where the mothers did not know

[1] See Vol. II, Part II.

how to deal with their children. This is in contrast with the close links between grandparents and parents in rural regions steeped in tradition.

Algeria is a country with a population of 10–11 million inhabitants, some of whom follow tribal customs while others have adopted European customs, especially in the towns. A difference can be seen in the practice of breast-feeding. In the towns artificial feeding is widespread among the natives, and although during the war some of the powdered milk distributed to the natives was diverted to the black market, some did use it to feed their children. In the country districts artificial feeding is practically unknown. The Algerian population has more than doubled during the last century, and whereas the absence of birth control has been offset by the enormous infant mortality, with modern medicine, this mortality has declined considerably. Algeria has begun to be unable to feed the whole population, and there is a drift towards the cities. Families have become disunited where the father has gone to work in France. He usually sends home his wages, but sometimes is away for long periods and forgets he has a family.

Social and family relationships: parents' personality. One problem worth notice is that of maternal anxiety which, in a modern society, can be allayed by talking with the paediatrician or the family doctor. In Algeria, with a more primitive culture, there is a tendency to give a name to a danger, as if the fact of naming the danger diminished it. The belief in genies gives rise to various customs, for instance, a child with conjunctivitis has a necklace put round its neck; when a mother has lost several of her children, her next baby is placed on an abandoned tomb and prayers are said so that the danger be turned away. It is dangerous to fight superstitions without replacing them with a more rational belief, but to do so, is a long and very difficult process.

Differences between cultural patterns, for example between Finland and the U.S.A., are startling in respect of family relationships. Someone coming from Finland might consider that the children in the United States were shockingly badly brought up, with an interesting cultural reluctance on the part of the parents to exercise authority. Parents in America appear to be reluctant to stand up for their beliefs. This may be because, as newcomers to the country, they want to become Americanized as soon as possible. Another point of difference is that the husband in the U.S.A. takes an active part in the house, even to washing diapers and hanging them out to dry. The division of labour in the household is more human and equitable than would be found in Finland.

It appears to be true that when parents want their children to do something they have not done themselves, the relationship between parent and child is altered. The parent can no longer be the model for the child's behaviour, as in a stable, traditional society. Such parents could be said to act like the lower-class nurse of the upper-class child: they feed, dress and educate their children as they were not fed, dressed or educated themselves. It is a conspicuous feature of undergraduate universities in the Middle West, that parents at university functions are dressed much worse than their children. It is impossible for such a father to be a model for the children; often he does not speak the language correctly. There is also a change of class, or from rural to city life. This phenomenon is also true of the countries of the Near East and South-East Asia where the children are becoming westernized. The child becomes master, because when the parent ceases to be the model, he cannot be master.

The child's need to have a model is shown by the way he creates a model if one does not exist. This is a parental function which exists of itself, and the child's imaginary father may be different from the real father. If they approximate to each other, the real father will have real authority, but if not, difficulties will arise.

Among the rural population of Norway, the father is the head of the family; three generations live together, the head of the family, his son, and his son's family. In the towns a generation ago, the father played the same role as in the country, but now the family is smaller, they live in smaller houses and flats, there is no domestic help and the father has to help run the house. With loss of autocracy there is increase in comradeship, a tendency to regard the family as a group of friends.

However, the opinion which the child has of the authority of the father depends mainly on the opinion generally accepted in the social structure to which they belong. In Algeria where the family is patriarchal, the child would not dare to criticize his father, or, if he does, he feels guilty. The father, even when absent, remains the supreme authority for the family, less because of his own personality than because of the cultural pattern.

The development of equality between boys and girls, attending the same schools, receiving the same professional training, has made girls become conscious that marriage is not necessarily their only security. Fathers and mothers have now a more equal voice in the home and the children understand this.

RECENT STUDIES OF CHILD DEVELOPMENT IN FRANCE

Irène Lézine

THE *Laboratoire de Psychobiologie de l'Enfant*, instituted in Paris by Professor Henri Wallon in 1926, and the *Service d'Etudes Génétiques*, under the direction of Professor R. Turpin, began to work together in 1942 on a joint research project on twins. In order to establish diagnostic norms a number of sets of uniovular and binovular twins were observed from the first weeks of life, so that the individual patterns of growth might be followed and the importance of the different periods of growth be determined. For this purpose a scale of tests for babies was devised, based on the work of Gesell, Bühler, Cattell, and others.

The scale was standardized in the big hospitals of Paris, in nine day-nurseries of the Public Assistance Department of the XIIIe and XIXe *Arrondissements*, in nursery schools, in Kindergartens of the *Habitations Bon Marché* (working-class housing estates), in a school employing an 'activities' method, and in four other types of school with methods varying from those of the Montessori tradition to others of more recent origin. Over the same period of time, children belonging to families in well-to-do circumstances were visited regularly for several years. Altogether, our norms were established on a sample of 1,500 children.

The *Centre d'Hygiène mentale*, of which Dr. Yves Porc'her is Director, entrusted to Mme. Brunet the development of a consultation service, including neurological, psychological and physiological examinations, for the early detection of behaviour disturbances in very small children. Mme. Brunet worked in a Health Centre in the XIVe *Arrondissement*, mainly with working-class families, and I myself worked in an Infant Welfare Centre at Puteaux.

At the same time Mme. Brunet and M. Zazzo, the present Director of the *Laboratoire de Psychobiologie de l'Enfant*, got together the group of young parents, who were all studying at the *Institut National d'Etude du Travail et d'Orientation Professionnelle* and at the *Institut de Psychologie*, who comprised the group of 'highly educated' parents mentioned in our reports.

During the first year of the inquiry, about twenty of these young psychologists were asked to write down in detail anything they noticed about the behaviour of their own children, and these observations were used as a control in testing the other groups. We were able to make regular examinations of these babies, and to film them in their normal surroundings.

During the second year the parents, by then used to this technique, took part in the observation of early imitative action on the part of the baby, his behaviour in front of a mirror, his awareness of self in various experimental situations, his language, the use of his own name, and so on.

In the third year we undertook a more theoretical study of attitudes to, or methods of, upbringing, as described in classical works concerning early childhood. The group employed a questionnaire, previously used by Mlle. Xydias and M. Clément to compare different regions in Europe. The questionnaire dealt with attitudes towards feeding, cleanliness, swaddling and matters of this sort.

In the following year there was an inquiry into relations between parents and children, as to whether, for example, the parents' preferences for their children determined the child's preference for its parents. The results are shortly to be published in the review *Enfance*. The group studied was made up of thirty-seven girls and thirty-four boys of from 15 months to 6 years of age, the average age being 3 years. It was seen how far the early care given to the child by the mother or father can have a determining influence on the child's preference later on, e.g., the more the father looked after the child in early years, the more there was a possibility of fixation on the part of the child. The role of the father in the children's play, which the group studied, also had an influence on this.

In the following year the group undertook the current research project and at the same time directed their attention more particularly towards family discipline, scolding, and punishment for disobedience. In addition to the twenty families of 'psychologist' parents, there are in the 126 families belonging to the 'better-educated' group of parents, ninety-two boys and ninety-two girls who are under observation from their earliest months up to 6 years. In particular, the stability of the development quotient in the $3\frac{1}{2}$- to 5-year period is being studied.

I have personally continued to specialize in work on young twins, and now have under observation fifty-five pairs, which I have studied from the age of 3 months up to 3 years. Mme. Brunet has specialized in problems of child-rearing, which may be brought to Infant Welfare Centres (Well Baby Clinics).

Comparison between Day-Nursery and Home Environment. It is common knowledge that the child brought up in a day-nursery, without toys and with inadequate staff, shows a significant retardation in comparison with the child brought up at home, even if he is taken home at the end of the day by his mother. In day-nurseries, a considerable backwardness in walking, cleanliness and talking, and in certain writing tests, is noticeable. We also found that children in this group, with a development quotient in many cases well below 90, quickly caught up on their backwardness when moved into a favourable environment.

This first observation was followed by a comparison of the mental development in working-class and well-to-do families: 149 children at health centres for working-class people, and sixty-four children from families in well-to-do circumstances, were studied, and at the same time the parents were asked about problems of upbringing and difficulties that they had encountered in rearing their children. In both groups there were no great difficulties among the children of less than 12 to 15 months old, who were being brought up by their parents. Difficulties increased between 15 and 30 months, and those which coincided with the various landmarks in the child's growth, were particularly numerous. Many more problems were found in families in better circumstances than in the working-class families. One might conclude that this difference, which was quite remarkable, was due to the fact that the better-off mothers were perhaps more observant and more prepared to answer questions: that the working-class mothers were more shy and less able to talk about their problems. However, we were not inquiring specifically into particular problems; our task was only to study the child's behaviour. The mothers did not know why we were there; they supposed us to be part of the permanent staff of the Health Centre, and were quite ready to confide their stories to us, and to ask for advice. Furthermore, we were only noting down the frequency of the problems which arose in these different environments. The better-off mothers had considerable anxieties as to how much food to give to the child and about the child's behaviour at meal-times. They asked questions about regularity of hours of sleep, behaviour and posture while asleep, and so on. We found toilet-training problems, tantrums and opposition to parents much more frequently in the better educated group, who had no clear notions about training. In fact the greatest confusion reigned with regard to what should or should not be done about the children.

Development Quotient in three Social Environments. The working-class group (see Table A) was composed of urban skilled workers, and, as shown, 80 per cent of the fathers were older than the mothers. At the Health Centre we were dealing especially with first-born children, but some of the families ranged from one to seven children. There were forty-three girls studied in this group and thirty-seven boys.

TABLE A

	Working-class Groups		Teachers, Artists, Psychologists, etc.		Engineers, Doctors, etc.	
	Average	Range	Average	Range	Average	Range
Average age of mothers	26	18–40	28	20–37	29	
Average age of fathers	27	18–51	28	20–39	32	
Fathers older than mothers	80%		35%		73%	
Average number of children per family	1 approx.	1–7	fewer		fewer	
Number of girls	43					
Number of boys	37					
Birth weight of girls	3.4 kg.	2.6–4.6	3.4 kg.	1.6–4.3	3.4 kg.	2.6–4.3
Birth weight of boys	3.5 kg.	2.6–4.6	3.43 kg.	2.6–4.6	3.43 kg.	1.6–4.6
First tooth—girls	6 mths.		6 mths.		6 mths.	
First tooth—boys	7 mths.		7 mths.		7 mths.	
Walking—girls	12-13 mths.		13 mths.		13 mths.	
Walking—boys	13 mths.		13 mths.		13 mths.	
First word—girls	8-9 mths.		8-9 mths.		8-9 mths.	
First word—boys	10-11 mths.		10 mths.		10 mths.	
Development quotient—girls	110	80–150	105	90–125	105	90–125
Development quotient—boys	102	80–124	100	83–103	100	83–103
Average salary			50–60,000		100,000+	
Fathers working			100%		100%	
Mothers working			80%		26%	

The families from the better educated circles were in two groups: one included school and university teachers, psychologists, artists, and so on, with an average salary of from 50,000 to 60,000 francs; and the other, engineers, doctors, and businessmen with salaries of over 100,000 francs. All the 'educated' fathers were working, as were 80 per cent of the mothers in the first group but only 26 per cent in the second. In the first of these groups, 40 per cent of the mothers were older and 25 per cent equal in age to the father, in contrast to the working-class families, where 80 per cent of the fathers were older. In the second group (engineers, doctors, etc.) only 10 per cent of the mothers were older and 17 per cent the same age. It seems that 'intellectuals' marry later and have fewer children than the other groups.

The developmental data in the three groups show little difference: any superiority there may be is in favour of the girls, which is, of course, well known, particularly in talking. But what happens later?

Long Term Follow-up. After a follow-up extending over several years, the interesting fact emerged that children in the group of families with a higher standard of education, showed an uninterrupted progression of the developmental quotient.[1] Table B shows that the

[1] When other tests are introduced this is not strictly a 'developmental quotient'.

boys developed more slowly (with a greater variety in the results), whereas the girls were ahead (particularly in verbal tests), up to the age of 4; later, the boys outstripped them. In the working-class group, stable development was found in the best cases, but there were rather spectacular regressions.

TABLE B

	Intellectual Group		School A		School B		School C	
	Boys	Girls	Average	Range	Average	Range	Average	Range
Number in the Group	20	20						
D.Q. at 12 months	100	100						
D.Q. at 2 years	102	104						
D.Q. at 3 years	102	109						
D.Q. at 4 years	105	111	100		85	75–126	106	100–112
D.Q. at 5 years	120	115	109	90–115	94	90–122	108	92–119
D.Q. at 6 years			116	90–150	87	84–123	115	89–150
D.Q. at 7 years			121	104–154	89	87–120	117	90–156

D.Q. = Development Quotient

A comparison was made between the pupils at some 'modern' schools. Of the three schools shown in Table B, 75 per cent of the parents of the pupils attending School 'A' were businessmen, bankers, or members of the better-paid professions, families with a higher standard of living; 30 per cent of the parents of those at School 'B' belonged to the lower-paid professions and 70 per cent were of the working-class; while with regard to 'C', 98 per cent of the parents belonged to the liberal professions. School 'B' had the best material equipment, the best lighting and hygienic conditions.

The regression noted in the 'B' group was very remarkable, and was most noticeable in the verbal aspects of the test.

A Study of Twins. A study of twins in four environments showed a fall in the average developmental quotient in the poorest environment (see Table C). In environment No. I, living conditions were wretched, and there was a very high percentage of unemployed or alcoholic fathers. No. II were artisans in a small way and semi-skilled craftsmen, with very low wages, living in two badly-furnished rooms. No. III were artisans, but with slightly higher wages of about 50,000 francs, and living in a three-roomed apartment or a little house in a suburb. No. IV were well-to-do parents, the fathers being businessmen or fully-trained engineers. The variations in the development quotient are very remarkable.

More remains to be said about twins, and close contact is being maintained with all these groups. We have been in touch with the 'intellectual' group regularly since 1946; Mme. Brunet continues to run a Health Centre at Courbevoie amongst the industrial working-class group; and one of the psychologists from the Research Centre goes regularly to the country where she is able to follow up 420 school children from the ages of 4 to 14 and also to see their younger brothers and sisters.

TABLE C.—A Study of Non-Identical Twins in Four Environments

	I	II	III	IV
Family Income	very low	Low	50,000 fr.	High
Number of rooms per family	1	2	3	Over 3
Average number of children per family	5	4	4	—
Average weight of boys at 12 months		9,600 gm.	10,800 gm.	11,300 gm.
Average weight of girls at 12 months		8,800 gm.	8,350 gm.	9,800 gm.
Average Development Quotient at 12 months	89	90	90	90
Average Development Quotient at 3 years	87	90	93	100

DISCUSSION

The inquiry clearly shows the importance of the family environment up to the age of 2 years. All the children made steady progress up to this age, while they remained, as in fact they did, in the care of their own family; but from the moment the child comes more into contact with the outside world, his environment changes, and his social surroundings begin to have an ever-increasing importance.

The conclusion from this is that, provided the conditions of life are comparable in the first years of life, differences in the cultural environment do not seem to be so very important.

The use of tests to bridge the gap between the infant development scales and intelligence tests for older children presents a big statistical problem to psychologists. The figures given in the inquiry have been in general only very rough, and very little importance should be attached to their actual level. But in spite of their lack of accuracy they show that there was a regression in one of the environments studied and a steady progress in another, though this could also be explained by the children's reaction to the tests themselves.

With regard to the tests used, studies in the United States have shown that intelligence tests were developed on middle-class samples by the middle-class for the middle-class. Tests using a middle-class

45

type of thought process will penalize members of the working-classes, especially by the use of a particular kind of vocabulary. In their own vocabulary, working-class people might do very much better.

The cultural resources of the environment—the number of objects, such as books and other sources of stimulation—also affect test results, and it has been suggested that among minority groups and in some cases among primitive people living in touch with civilization, a child, as he gets older, may decide for himself whether it is important to learn or whether it is not important. At one time psychologists used to claim that American Negro children were very bright when they were little, but not when they were older; but it was found that this was not true of Negro children who moved north, and that the phenomenon was related to the child's expectation of being able to use his learning.

When seeking reasons for the difference in children's progress in the various economic and social groups, it is interesting to study the importance of nutrition. In the United States it has been shown that very poorly nourished children might have a very mediocre intelligence or developmental quotient, which would alter after several months of proper feeding. The conditions of undernourishment were, of course, extreme—not just a question of vitamin B or C deficiency. There is a tendency among most people at a poverty level of subsistence to feed the baby more liberally than the older children, so it is important to know how far the regression observed among the very poorest group was due to the older children receiving a smaller proportion of the available food.

A group of children, specially studied in a day-nursery, showed very poor development, but it improved when they were removed to a better environment in a nursery school. Their earlier regression was very considerable, because they had lived in good family conditions during their early months.

This observation was made on children whose mothers were working in a factory with a day-nursery where they could leave the children in the morning and take them home in the evening. Though the children were not completely removed from family life, practically everything was done for them at the day-nursery, and they actually had very little real contact with their mothers.

When the children were 2½ the mothers could no longer leave them in the day-nurseries, and they were sent to a nursery school, of which one was attached to each group of houses in a housing project. Here the staff were much better trained, and the nursery school teacher played with the children; but she did not wash or feed them, so that their mothers had much more to do with them. This is one explanation of their faster rate of development later.

In the day-nurseries studied, in very poor districts, the children had no play equipment or toys at all. They were kept in their cots and only taken out for about half an hour during the day, the reason being that there was only one person to look after them. Thus the regression noticed corresponded with unfavourable conditions of life, but with better conditions development not only caught up to the right level but often went beyond it. A deeper study of the main factors in this change has not yet been made.

PARENTS' ATTITUDES AND THE BEHAVIOUR OF YOUNG CHILDREN

Irène Lézine

A QUALIFIED PSYCHOLOGIST had already been working for some time in each field of research before we began this study. Pierrette Brochay and Hilda Santucci were in the country with two ethnologists; Odette Brunet and Marianne LeGuay were in the working-class neighbourhood of Courbevoie, a suburb of Paris; and I myself was also in Paris, studying the better-educated families with M. Massé, an ethnologist. In the country we carried out the inquiry by means of interviews, as it was difficult to make tests because we were not well-known to the families; but in the towns the children of the working-class families were tested, and their parents were visited several times; and of the more educated group, which was the best known to us, not only the children, but to some extent, the parents, were tested.

The urban working-class group. These families were fairly well-off, and except for their poor housing, not strictly speaking typical of working-class families in France; but their living quarters lacked light and space, and the sanitary conditions were bad. Many families had no running water laid on and were obliged to fetch water from up or down one or two flights of stairs.

The rural group. The country families were not particularly representative because of sampling difficulties. The group included rich farmers and the agricultural labourers working on their farms, whose living conditions were very different from those of their employers. There were thus two distinct standards of living in the group.

The better-educated group. Our conclusions cannot be applied generally to the better-educated Parisian families, but only to those few in which one of the parents at least has studied psychology. The group we studied also had rather poor housing, but the standard of living varied greatly. Some lived three in one room, other families had a little house in a suburb, and others lived in one very poorly furnished hotel room. Most of them complained of their housing conditions. This group is discussed in more detail on p. 49.

48

The upbringing of the children. In all three groups there were no very clear-cut ideas about bringing up children, but the working-class families on the whole had a stricter attitude than the others with regard to discipline and training. This, according to M. Chombart de Lauwe, as well as in our opinion, can be explained by their living conditions: the workers are themselves accustomed to strict time-tables, cramped surroundings, and hard working conditions. Their states of weariness and tension are reflected in their impatience towards their children, in relation to whom they showed considerable severity and emotional instability; that is, swift and sudden changes from tenderness to disciplinary action.

In the more educated group the attitude might be called 'excessively liberal': the parents were aware that there were many problems in bringing up children and this knowledge strengthened their tendency not to interfere. The mothers gave the impression of being afraid of intervening, of preferring to allow their children to do whatever they wanted rather than take action and give rise to conflicts between themselves and the children.

In the country the attitude was very liberal, but the children were much less often in contact with adults; they enjoyed more space and possibilities for amusement than the children in the other groups.

Features common to all groups. Walking started in all three groups at 13 months, two months earlier than in previous observations of children. Most of the children did not, before learning to walk, go through the various crawling stages described by Gesell in his study of child development. The reasons for this are not clear, but it is possible that a child who is placed at an early age in a play-pen learns, by clinging on to the bars of the pen, to stand earlier than the child who has no support within reach.

In toilet-training, not much advantage appeared to be gained from trying to train a child before the age of 12 months. Other things being equal, in the working-class and better-educated circles the children did not acquire clean habits any earlier, no matter at what age the training was started. Below a certain degree of maturity training seemed to be useless.

We found that children had a greater tendency to suck their thumbs when weaning had been sudden or very early.

THE BETTER-EDUCATED GROUP

In this group most of the parents were teachers. All the fathers, and all except four of the mothers, were working or had once worked. Their way of living was modest, the family budget being rarely higher

E   49

than 80,000 francs. From the cultural point of view they were homogeneous, all having had secondary education and courses in psychology. Their families had lived for about two generations in provincial towns, and in most cases the parents came from different provinces. The average age of the parents was 30 for fathers and 28 for mothers, and 45 per cent to 50 per cent of the mothers were older than the fathers. It would be interesting to know whether this would be true of teachers and psychologists in other countries. The general average for France is that the father is four years older than the mother. We noticed that the wives who were older than their husbands were in many cases the dominating partner, exercising more control over the children, managing the family budget, and taking all decisions relating to the children. Maternal domination emerged very strongly in our study of this group.

We worked with these families for several years to find out what additional information could be obtained by means of a questionnaire and to what extent the questionnaire would agree with previous observations. One interesting result was that the ethnological questionnaire established a large number of factors which had eluded observation in previous inquiries. It was also proved to be an advantage to have these families visited by different interviewers or research workers.

Attitudes towards the upbringing of children in the better-educated group. On the whole, the mothers closely followed the advice given by handbooks on modern child care. This applied to breast and bottle-feeding, a liquid diet followed by the introduction of solid foods, and so on. There was great variety in the parents' ideas about rearing their children. We were struck by the very large number of children who had difficulties, or problems. This fact does not, perhaps, emerge sufficiently clearly from the questionnaire, for although our statistics suggest that the children in this group cried more, both day and night, sucked their thumbs more, and more often had obsessional habits than any of the others, this is not sufficiently marked for them to be classed as 'difficult' children.

As the children had been under observation for a long time, we were able to take note of many problems of which the parents themselves were not fully aware. In particular, 65 per cent of the children in this group were difficult over their food, systematically refusing it, vomiting, or making scenes at table which were very upsetting both for the parents and the children.

In most cases the mothers did not attempt a systematic toilet-training, but in spite of this tolerant attitude there seemed to be quite a large number of children who went through very difficult periods of opposition, perhaps more severe than in the other groups. Obsessional habits such as thumb-sucking, affection for certain objects, and so on, were observed in 60 per cent of the children. It is an open question whether this exaggerated attachment to objects may not be due to the parents' own attitude, since they themselves ascribed great importance to the child's earliest possessions, to the custom of making a first present to the child at its birth, to the selection of presents and the use of the colour considered correct for a girl or a boy—points much less noticeable in the other groups.

Scoldings and punishments were much less severe in this group; not only did the parents interfere less with the behaviour of their children, but also the kind of punishment meted out was very different from that used in the other groups. Isolation was imposed as a punishment in this group only, the child being taken to another room, away from the scene of the conflict. Some parents thought that the child probably looked on this as much worse than smacking. In a study of the attitudes of parents, we found that in this group punishments differed considerably according to the child's sex. While the mothers were much more strict with their sons with regard to their behaviour in social and family life and towards other people, they were more impatient with their little daughters. With older children five different kinds of punishment were used. First, explanations, reasoning, persuasion; secondly, firmness, a show of authority without explanation; thirdly, isolating the child; fourthly, irony, joking, ridicule, teasing; and fifthly, smacks and blows. Both fathers and mothers were equally strict with boys and used the same kind of punishment to the same extent, but where girls were concerned, explanation, reasoning and persuasion were used by the fathers but very rarely by the mothers. It would seem that mothers did not waste much time on their daughters, trying to explain what they had done right or wrong; they wanted to settle matters more quickly. Irony, joking and humour were not used with daughters, either by the father or the mother, but smacks and blows were more common with both parents, particularly the father. It was evident, furthermore, that sometimes the parents were more attached to a son than to a daughter.

This greater attachment to the son was also shown in another small experiment. We asked the fathers and mothers to define the qualities they thought the most important for their children to possess, and to list the virtues and faults that they had observed in them. In both cases the mothers were much more demanding and strict with their daughters, and the fathers less exacting; the fathers thought daughters were easier to manage and had fewer faults. Conversely, the mothers were more indulgent towards the boys and found them easier to manage. With boys, mothers attached more importance than fathers to moral qualities and to affection; and fathers attached more importance to intellectual, physical and social qualities. With daughters, mothers wanted more in respect of intellectual and moral qualities, and fathers were keener on sociability and affection. For instance, the mothers listed intelligence, independence, courage, perseverance, and frankness as the most important qualities for girls; whereas fathers spoke more about affection, gentleness, power of observation and sensitivity. The differences between the parents were much less as regards the qualities expected of a boy, and as far as faults were concerned there was agreement; the most frequent faults of character in boys were said to be anger and disobedience, and in girls, obstinacy and selfishness.

To sum up, various questions arise: why were these children more difficult than the children in the other groups? Perhaps the fact that the mothers tended to be older and more dominating than the fathers may be one of the reasons. The mothers were more anxious, and the living conditions may have added to the trouble. Teachers tend to have full time-tables, which make them tense and irritable. When the fathers came home after coping all day with big classes and too heavy a programme, they found it difficult to be patient with their own children. Furthermore, their working conditions were not entirely satisfactory, and they lacked security. In most cases they were vocational guidance counsellors, studying in Paris, and did not yet know where they would eventually be posted; and their own insecurity tended to react on the children. Even if they would have liked to give time to their children, they were overloaded with professional duties, and had too little time to spare.

These parents often complained of the lack of properly equipped day-nurseries and nursery schools in their neighbourhood, and that the nursery schools they would have chosen were overcrowded. Many of them had to have their children looked after at home by people who they did not think were suitably qualified, which meant that they were having to pay somebody with whose ideas they often disagreed, to look after their children.

To end on a personal note, I should like to emphasize the value and interest of working in a team of psychologists, ethnologists and doctors, when studying the life and development of young children.

DISCUSSION

Early Toilet-training. A distinction had been drawn between walking, which is a stage of natural development, and clean habits, which result from training; and it had also been said that very early toilet-training did not appear to be an effective way of achieving clean habits, and that its results were no better than with training begun later. But in exceptional cases, children can be successfully toilet-trained from the age of three weeks, so that it is in fact possible to teach these habits, although some may believe that to do so is quite useless.

Perhaps the greatest contribution to mental hygiene is to have a service for supplying clean napkins to mothers who are overwhelmed by the problem of doing their washing in their tiny rooms. A great deal of tension could be avoided if this question were solved. In present conditions, many parents understandably wish their children to be clean as soon as possible.

No study has yet been made of any connection between feeding problems and toilet-training, but such a study should be possible. Other factors enter into sphincter control; the influence of the environment is more often focussed on clean habits by day than by night. The latter, like walking, is more closely connected with the natural development pattern, except in the case of a disturbed child with whom enuresis may be a sort of semi-conscious protest.

United Kingdom

BACKGROUND
TO CHILD DEVELOPMENT PATTERNS
IN THE UNITED KINGDOM. (I)

D. R. MacCalman

LIKE DR. BOUTONIER and Dr. Jackson, with regard to French and American children, I could say that the typical British child both does and does not exist. Since hearing the United States and French accounts of development patterns, I feel that the British child is different from his counterpart in these countries—a difference which grows stronger as age increases. But, as in France, it is impossible to talk about clear-cut and specific developmental patterns which are peculiar to Great Britain alone. There are, moreover, in England, Scotland, Wales, and Northern Ireland, distinct cultural groups, with differing environments, religions and ideals, and different speech. Local customs, social backgrounds and developmental influences differ. Even the cities such as Leeds, are not by any means homogeneous, socially, racially, or traditionally. For example there is a higher Jewish proportion of the population in Leeds than in the city of New York. The cultural pattern differs not only from north to south but also from east to west; but my remarks are confined to Yorkshire, and in particular to Leeds, and even to a single area of that city.

A good deal of my experience of early development and its influence on personality was gained in Aberdeen, although I am not myself an Aberdonian, and my views may be affected by what I learned there. However, there is a resemblance between Leeds and Aberdeen, between Yorkshire and Buchan, and the trilogy of Lewis Grassic Gibbon describes with clinical accuracy the Mearns, that is the district round about Aberdeen, and its folk, in a way in which, but for the difference in dialect, Phyllis Bentley or Winifred Holtby might describe Yorkshire.

I would like to give you a short extract from one of the stories of Lewis Grassic Gibbon (12):

'She'd had nine of a family in her time, Mistress Menzies, and brought the nine of them up, forbye—some near by the scruff of the

54

neck, you would say. They were sniftering and weakly, two-three of the bairns, sniftering in their cradles to get into their coffins; but she'd shake them to life, and dose them with salts and feed them up till they couldn't but live. And she'd plonk one down—finishing the wiping of the creature's neb or the unco dosing of an ill bit stomach or the binding of a broken head—with a look on her face as much as to say "Die on me now and see what you'll get!" . . . But feint the much time to look or to listen had Margaret Menzies of Tocherty toun. Day blinked and Meg did the same, and was up, out of her bed, and about the house, making the porridge and rousting the bairns, and out to the byre to milk the three kye, the morning growing out in the east and a wind like a hail of knives from the hills. Syne back to the kitchen again she would be, and catch Jock, her eldest, a clour in the lug that he hadn't roused up his sisters and brothers; and rouse them herself, and feed them and scold, pull up their breeks and straighten their frocks, and polish their shoes and set their caps straight. "Off you get and see you're not late," she would cry, "and see you behave yourselves at the school. And tell the Dominie I'll be down the night to ask him what the mischief he meant by leathering Jeannie and her not well."

'They'd cry "Ay, Mother," and go trotting away, a fair flock of the creatures, their faces red-scoured. Her own as red, like a meikle roan mare's, Meg'd turn at the door and go prancing in; and then at last, by the closet-bed, lean over and shake her man half-awake. "Come on, then, Willie, it's time you were up." '

You will note how forceful and authoritative, how robust and Elizabethan is this mother, but how warm in her protection and her affection for her children. Note, too, how she reserved the right of punishment for herself and rushes to their defence whenever anybody else, such as this school master, dares to punish her children. The whole story illustrates behaviour of this type: how vigorously she defended one daughter accused of stealing, swept a son into marriage with a girl that he had got into trouble, supported her daughter who wanted to live with but not marry her lover. The *dénouement* comes when this mother, so upright, always so proper and well-doing, in her own old age explains to her scandalized children that she never quite got round to marrying Willie. You will have noted how tender and forgiving she was, however, to this weak, alcoholic and ne'er-do-well marriage partner. In short no one could fail to see how her love burned warmly through this rugged exterior.

In Yorkshire, too, there is a similar warmth. The shopkeeper or tramcar conductor will call you 'Luv', irrespective of sex or age or social status; and surely there can be fewer more hospitable communities. The sheer enjoyment of neighbourliness cannot be better illustrated than in a Yorkshire pub or at a cricket match or on a bus trip to Blackpool. The resemblance between those two areas is such that you might easily mistake one for the other, and justifiably so, for the creatures of the Yorkshire dales and the mill towns are 'canny, slow and quiet' like the folk of the Mearns; and no more than a meagre living has ever been wrung from the soil, 'all fyled wi' clay, and dour wi' chuckies'. Life in such parts is known to be a grim, relentless struggle, and there is a fierce contempt for those who wilt under the strain. Here I might quote the Scottish poet, Robert Louis Stevenson, addressing the man who protests against grinding poverty and the inhospitality of Nature. He says to him:

> 'What you would like's a palace ha',
> Or Sunday parlour dink and braw,
> Wi' a' things ordered in a row
> By denty ladies.
> The shoon ye colt, the life ye lead,
> Ithers will heir when aince ye're dead;
> They'll heir your tasteless bite of bread,
> An' find it sappy;
> They'll to your dulefu' house succeed
> An' there be happy.'

Upbringing, as you can imagine, in such parts of this island was traditionally designed to fit the child for a hard life. A parent, and particularly a mother, faced a perpetual struggle between her tender feelings, her happiness in her children, and her belief that it was her duty to extract implicit and patient obedience, uncomplaining acceptance of frustration, and faith that there is a reason and a purpose in adversity. One can hear long generations of mothers saying to their fractious children:

> 'My bonnie man, the world, it's true,
> Was made for neither me nor you;
> It's just a place to wrasle through,
> As Job confessed to't,
> And aye the best that we can do
> Is mak' the best o't.'

And when you see the mean little streets and mean little houses of Leeds, with the sky hidden by black, greasy smoke for much of the year, perhaps you will not be surprised at this tradition. When you realize that tall chimneys have replaced tall trees; that clear streams have become grey canals; that green pastures are now grimy pavements and cobbled streets, perhaps you will understand that that robustness, that coarseness even, must be cultivated if any satisfaction is to be found in life.

While this may be the traditional background to child-rearing in Yorkshire, a warmer influence has blown upon it with increasing force for the last two generations. The young mother finds life, in many ways, less grim than did her grandmother. There is more money and fuller employment. The working-classes can be said to be in command of the employer-employee relationship. It is no longer necessary for a worker to fear dismissal for what might be called a leisurely attitude towards work, or an unskilled performance. The hard task-master soon finds himself begging for mercy. Even economic blizzards have lost their crippling power, for, in Leeds at least, a recession in one industry is followed by a transfer of the redundant worker to another. The Welfare State has feverishly increased its responsibilities until no one is ill-clad or hungry, and no one experiences real want or poverty.

Fathers and mothers, too, have been educated in a kindlier way. The 400-year old Grammar School may struggle to maintain its standards of hard work and harder punishment, but, for the first time in its history, the Headmaster is not a Minister of the Church. Throughout the State schools an altogether easier and more permissive existence is enjoyed by the pupils. The recognition of individual differences in ability means that punishment follows unruly behaviour rather than scholastic failure. Authoritarianism gradually fades from the scene and awe-stricken respect for elders and betters is being replaced by a friendlier co-operation between pupil and teacher. Classes are still too large and many schools have dingy and unattractive buildings, but there is no doubt that children enjoy their tasks in a way which was hardly possible formerly.

All this has, in my opinion, a significant effect upon the parents when they, in turn, come to bring up their own children. They have had no example or precept set them of a dominating and demanding attitude towards the young, the weak and the helpless. On the whole they have enjoyed their contact with those in authority and have felt free and unafraid. Children, they feel, have a right to happiness and bright childhood memories. There is no doubt that they would rather be loved than respected by their children and that they strive for companionship rather than slavish obedience from them.

Here I would like to state a personal opinion: that I am greatly comforted with what I see in the generation of young people now having their first babies. To a large extent they balance the two previous generations—their grim, stern grandparents and their over-protective, over-anxious and bewildered parents. This generation shows, at least, a welcome tendency to calmness and naturalness, to intelligent understanding and knowledge, combined at the same time with healthy and unfevered emotion.

Two other factors have brought this warmer and more balanced climate of opinion into the Yorkshire dales. The first is the greatly improved and expanded statutory provisions for the health and welfare of mothers and infants. In Leeds you may see a church which, significantly, has been converted into a maternity and child welfare clinic—a conversion which indicates something more than the great shortage of suitable premises for such organizations. Health, indeed, may be said to be the new religion. 'And a good thing too, much better than the worship of Mammon', as one of my staff said to me when I pointed this out to him.

From the moment when she conceives, every mother who can be persuaded, is cosseted and cared for: from the moment of birth every child is treated as a jewel of great price. A great army of doctors, maternity nurses, physiotherapists, Public Health and paediatric nurses sweep the mother along on the wave of their enthusiastic demand that no trouble or expense should be spared to give the baby his right to the enjoyment of a robust existence, as well as absence from disease and the expectation of survival. Nor is it considered sufficient to leave these high aspirations in the hands of professional experts, for much time and care is expended upon teaching the mother and in attempting to make her an expert in baby care, with almost professional knowledge and skill. Roberts, Corner and Davies, in their *Textbook for Health Visitors* (23), speak of the Health Visitor as 'the adviser in preventative medicine and health teacher to the families under her care and supervision.'

Here it should be admitted that until very recently the major attention has been paid to physical health and bodily welfare. Many of my psychiatric colleagues are highly critical of the neglect of the mental aspects of health. For my own part I am inclined to think that little time has been wasted. For one thing, mental hygiene, as we are experiencing now, is still in its own infancy and, for all the claims to the contrary, even a few years ago psychiatrists and psychologists had little to offer of positive or practical value to the normal mother with her normal child. A fine organization has been set up in this country, dealing with those aspects of mother and child which few dispute and which indeed the public demand as their right and their children's right. Nothing in this country is set up by the Government unless the people demand it, almost at the point of the sword. Nor has mental hygiene been entirely neglected, even though the practice of some of its principles is fortuitous and unwitted.

The mother has at least emerged as the important figure in the care of infants, and that reminds me of the story of the man who rushed out of an apartment house in New York, frantically signalled a taxi, jumped in, and told the driver to drive with all speed to the maternity hospital, explaining that it was a matter of life and death. The taxi-driver drove off with great sound and fury, but just as they got to the maternity hospital the embarrassed passenger had to tell him to go back for his expectant wife! Sometimes the mother and the child have been forgotten in our deliberations; but, perhaps unprompted by psychiatric teaching, separation of the mother and child is now frowned upon, and even paediatric hospitals are trying hard to catch up. Every effort is made to make the mother more confident and more expert in her handling of her baby. She is encouraged to be lavish with her affection and permissive in her training, and again her advisers have had little direct influence from mental hygienists. Rather, these advisers of the mother would disclaim, embarrassed, any knowledge of such abstruse and subtle intentions, and defend their teaching on the grounds of what they call 'sound common sense'. They are quite pleased, of course, when their techniques and practice are confirmed by mental health experts; perhaps mildly surprised at this unexpected evidence of good sense on the part of the psychiatrists; but that they are right they have never doubted. I need not enlarge upon their possible reaction to any advice which might not agree with their practice. We must realize that there will be marked resistance if any significant change in contemporary child-rearing practices is suggested in the interests of mental health. So far, no major change has been suggested, and this is perhaps why we are allowed to play some small part in the training of doctors and others concerned with maternal and child welfare.

I am tempted to speculate upon the possibility of this emphasis upon health having an adverse psychological effect upon mothers and children. If health is worshipped so eagerly, may not the acolytes become morbidly afraid of disease, or resentful and depressed when the ideal of athletic ebullience is not attained? Or what feelings of guilt may a mother suffer when her child dies or is handicapped or diseased? As a nation we may very well be selling our all for that pearl of great price, the healthy child, and some parents are going to find, or are already finding, that their sacrifices and their endeavours are fruitless. Nor are many parents able to console themselves nowadays with the belief that God gathers His most precious souls to be with Him in Paradise, undimmed by the cares and corruptions of a sinful world.

In the meantime, however, any such speculations upon the possible effect of a worship of health must remain speculations until sufficient time has elapsed to produce enough evidence for us to examine.

Another trend is the increasing uniformity and standardization of child-rearing practices as between one social class and another, and as between one part of the country and another. Time was when practice in cottage and castle showed wide differences; when it was possible to tell at a glance the baby of the rich, the poor and the middle-class parents. Not only was the dress more sumptuous and elaborate, the pram or baby carriage more elegant, the nursery and the nannie the prerogative of the upper classes, but the baby itself would show by its state of nutrition, by its cleanliness or lack of it, or by its physical development, the social status of its parents. Now, as a Director of a City Health Service recently remarked, one cannot possibly tell whether it is a miner's or a successful businessman's child, when it is undressed; and only at a guess when it is clothed and in its pram. Prams now tend to be handed down from one generation to another, or from family to family, among the professional classes and not, as formerly, among the manual working-class. You will see surprisingly smart and expensive prams parked outside the maternity and child welfare clinic in the slums.

The education of mothers about nutrition, through Health Visitors, maternity and child welfare clinics and other State assistance, has been surprisingly effective, even among the submerged tenth. As a result, rickets and other nutritional disorders have virtually disappeared, though one may still occasionally see what are known as 'Leeds legs'. Leeds legs were the typical bow legs of the rickety child that were so common two generations ago in big cities like Leeds, Glasgow, and Manchester.

Another indication of improved nutrition is given by the still-birth rate, which dropped in Leeds from 0·77 per thousand in 1930 to 0·37 in 1950. It is surprising to find that babies of all classes are fed in the same way, with the same foods and in the same proportions —that is, when they have finished breast-feeding or when they are artificially fed. The use of National Dried Milk is universally popular, although the Ministry of Food are a little embarrassed about this, because their care, as Civil Servants, is not to press its use, in case this should interfere with their ideal of breast-feeding for all.

Rations of vitamins such as cod-liver oil capsules, orange-juice, and so on, are available to every mother, whether rich or poor, and the consumption of cows' milk, at a later stage of the child's development, has increased to an enormous extent since before the recent war. Then there are preparations which are used almost universally—cereal foods prepared from wheat, oats, and so on.

There still remains one sharp distinction between one social class and another, and that is in the type and extent of living space. This is a burning social problem, which receives the highest priority in all political parties and in every succeeding Government. Politicians would not dare to give housing anything but the highest priority in men and materials, and in spite of this the people are still angry and dissatisfied with the rate of building. New hospitals, schools, and university departments must give way to houses for the people and plans for the former will perhaps remain neglected throughout our lifetime. There is an urgent need for new houses for those who have no roof of their own, or for those who live in the slums.

I recall hearing a paediatrician giving advice about the use of a play-pen to the mother of a hyper-active child. She was indignant, because the specialist did not realize that there was no room to put up a play-pen in the one living-room of her house in Leeds, the front door of which opened on to the pavement of a busy street; nor was there any backyard, for her neighbour's kitchen was where the backyard normally would be. Often you will see such a room so crammed with furniture that there is scarcely room to move, far less to set up a play-pen. One wonders why these rooms were built so small, but when the houses were first built, about the middle of the nineteenth century, they would not have seemed so small to the people who lived there, for they were really poor and had not enough money to buy furniture to overcrowd the houses. To-day the inhabitants are no longer poor in household goods and chattels, so that into this tiny space must go the gas or electric cooker, the water heater, the three-piece suite, the table, the sideboard and chairs, the pram, the television set and, of course, the human beings. Now these latter—the human beings—are the most easily movable and the children are frequently banished to play in the streets, except for mealtimes and bedtimes, and you can imagine that this contributes to juvenile delinquency. It adds, too, to the worries about pregnancies: a mother was asked how she managed in the space at her disposal, and she replied that she could just manage now with two children but had no idea what would happen if she had another.

Nor do these slum dwellers have any faith that better houses will come in the foreseeable future. Some of them have had their names registered with the local council for ten or fifteen years, and they can hardly believe that they will be allocated a house before they are too old to need it. In Leeds in 1949 there were roughly 154,000 houses: 90,000 were obsolescent, 56,000 were back-to-back houses. The oldest type of back-to-back houses, built before 1884, accounts for 16,000; an intermediate type, 8,000, and the newest type, 12,000.

16,000 remain from the pre-war slum clearance programme, ear-marked for demolition in 1934; with the result that repairs have been minimal for eighteen years, and in addition another 8,000 houses are now considered quite unfit for habitation. During the period 1946/51 inclusive, 443 houses have been demolished out of this 56,000.

There are no houses in Leeds without fresh water laid on indoors, but the oldest and the intermediate back-to-back houses are usually without internal sanitation. The oldest houses have a group of W.C.s to every eight houses, the more recent, a group to every six or even four houses. The newest type of back-to-back house may have its own sanitation, but outside the house; and where there is no internal sanitation, slops are either carried to the privy or, more conveniently, they are poured directly into the street drains.

So you can see that lack of living room, lack of space for children to grow, may have a significant effect upon both physical and mental development; though, of course, the conditions of the physical environment are not nearly so important as the climate of family relationship. This hungry desire, this longing for a house of one's own, big enough to bring up a family in, has its pathetic aspect in those few cases where it is granted. The splendid new house, so long dreamed of, may be on a housing estate which seems very remote to the family; they are banished from their friends to a so-called 'better' neighbourhood which, to begin with at least, they find chilly and remote. There may be none of the warm neighbourliness of the public house, the fish-and-chips shop, the stores and the picture house, and this throws the mother and children into an isolation which raises tension and dependency to a harmful degree. Quite a number return to the slums, even to worse conditions than they had left. I wonder whether our town planners are sufficiently aware of the benefits of neighbourliness in child-rearing.

BACKGROUND TO
CHILD DEVELOPMENT PATTERNS
IN THE UNITED KINGDOM. (II)

D. R. MacCalman

THERE IS a large gap in pre-natal mental hygiene, where fathers ought to be; the father is a figure of fun in many civilizations, although perhaps that is not such a serious thing in itself. I remember a cartoon in *The New Yorker*, in which you saw a very weedy and weak-looking little man, rather sub-human, standing in the corridor outside the delivery room in a maternity hospital; the nurse was opening the door with an expression of absolute astonishment on her face, holding out an infant and saying 'Congratulations, it's a baby!'

We fathers do not mind being figures of fun now and then, but being a father is really, or should be, a position of dignity and responsibility. It seems that in Leeds the role played by the father in the upbringing of the infant is very insignificant. In many cases he can be regarded as a displaced person, in the mysterious happenings of pregnancy and birth; and yet there is at the same time very strong evidence of the great emotional and moral support that enlightened and confident husbands can give to their wives at such times—if they know what is going on and are allowed to co-operate. It is generally supposed, in our country, that fathers have no wish or aptitude for child care, and yet this is strange, because the traditional idea of tender care is symbolized by the shepherd and his flock. In some primitive tribes, the care of the infant is entrusted to the father. An interesting fact which emerged from our inquiries before the Seminar, is that if the marriage is truly co-operative, and the wife actually knows what her husband's salary is and shares in any wage increase that may take place, then the father is allowed to take part in the rearing of his children. Where, on the other hand, the mother does not know, but only bitterly suspects what her husband's pay is, she does not allow him to have any part in the early rearing, at least, of her family. At a later stage she will make a bogey-man of the father, by saying 'You wait till Father comes home, then you will see what you will get.'

In many families the father has little influence on his baby, and his unco-operative attitude in turn may very gravely affect his wife's

63

state of mind. For this reason the need for education of both mothers and fathers, both boys and girls, is very important. Education of this kind must be simple and practical, and it needs a body of suitably trained people to carry it out. The health visitor, maternity and child welfare staffs, the family doctor, the regional psychiatrist with mental hygiene responsibilities and the voluntary bodies such as the Marriage Guidance Council, are all important in this respect. These aspects of mental hygiene lie beyond the bounds of medicine; responsibility for them rests not entirely with doctors but with those lay people whose co-operation is needed so very badly. Work of this type fosters the growth of preventive psychiatry, where 'the tentative ideas of to-day become the standard practice of respectable authority to-morrow.'

How do parents, and particularly mothers, actually feel about having a family? First, how would they feel about not having a family at all? It emerges from our inquiry that childlessness would have given rise to considerable anxiety in women of all classes. One or two of the professional class expressed this very strongly; one said 'I would have felt that my life had not been justified.' About a half would have wanted to adopt a child, if they were unable to have one of their own, although others, when questioned about adoption, said that they were afraid of bad heredity. Note the very strong belief that character and personality are mainly dependent upon inborn factors. Few parents consciously blame themselves if the child turns out badly in any way, but they look back through the family tree for an explanation in as remote a branch as they can find. Nor do parents really give themselves credit if the child develops satisfactorily: rather they feel that luck or Divine Providence has favoured them, and never do they see their own affection as a primary factor in the good result; the physical care, perhaps; the discipline, maybe; but the love and protection—never. There seems to be an important piece of information which we have failed to get across to the community, that affection is necessary: that it is as desirable for the child's development as vitamins or an adequate diet. It would be interesting to know why parents are so shy about showing affection overtly to their children?

The first child is usually very eagerly looked forward to, and a great sense of achievement is felt both by the mother and by the father. But pregnancy is often delayed, mostly for financial or housing reasons, or, in other words, young married couples tend to have a family as soon as they have a house of their own. The suggestion that international tension, fear of war and the consequent separation must be reckoned as a factor in delaying having a family may be true in certain cases, but I do not think it is very general.

The main factors are housing, space, and, of course, money. One health visitor summed up the general feeling as follows: 'Attitudes towards having the first child vary from pleasure in the majority, annoyance in the few who are pleasure-seekers or in business, dismay where it is essential for the woman to work although married, and panic and defiance among unmarried girls.'

Illness during pregnancy often causes both father and mother to regret it, and the immediate reaction of the mother after pregnancy is very often 'Never again', but this lasts for a short time only and she begins to look forward to having another child. The second pregnancy is looked forward to by the majority, who are influenced greatly by a sense of duty to the first child. Only children are believed to be under a great handicap; mothers will say that they are so easily spoiled, they are so lonely, they miss all the fun of having a playmate—and here you will note that the possibility of jealousy situations is almost completely repressed. I think that psychiatrists might do more to reassure those many women who have only one child, that that child need not necessarily grow up to be spoiled or mentally handicapped. The father often shares this idea, so that the first two children are usually wanted.

Until the second pregnancy marital relationships are good more often than not, and sexual intercourse is enjoyed; but thereafter a dramatic change takes place. In the lower income group, with few exceptions, the woman then dreads intercourse and pregnancy, and marital relationships may deteriorate quite markedly. Such mothers feel literally that there will be not enough food for another baby, not enough clothing, not enough living space; and this fear may be based to some extent on reality. For example, there was the mother living in the crowded back-to-back house who said, spontaneously, 'I can manage all right with two, but what will happen when another comes along?' The fear that there will not be enough money will not necessarily be based on the husband's wage but on the mother's memory perhaps, of unemployment and economic depression; or she may receive only a meagre percentage of her husband's wage, and many wives benefit in no way from a wage increase. Even some of those who get a fair share have quite a hard time managing, particularly when the economic situation is not stable.

So it is a common practice for women to go out to work, in order to supplement the family income, even although their children may be under 2 years old. The Public Health Department of Leeds has fifteen day-nurseries, with 800 places, of which 274 are reserved for babies under 2 years old. There are also four other licensed day-nurseries, and twenty-three registered child-minders who look after eighty-four children. This makes a total of just under 1,000 children who are being looked after at public expense, out of a yearly total of 9,000 births, and, of course, it does not include those looked after privately in their own families. Therefore, although many lower-class mothers would prefer to have three children, one, as they say, of each sex and another of either sex for luck, and some long for a big family, the vast majority have only two and very few have four.

Some unwanted pregnancies occur, to the surprise and annoyance of those who use birth control. Many attempt to terminate the pregnancy but only, as a rule, by the use of herbs and castor oil and pills and, of course, 'mother's ruin'—gin. The law strictly precludes any possibility of surgical termination, except where the mother's life or reason is in danger.

Among the university mothers, the size of family considered ideal is slightly higher; thus they may wish for two, three or six children, even, but it is doubtful whether all achieve the income level at which their ideal family is thought possible. Income tax and super-tax reduce professional salaries by about 50 per cent. In university circles £2,000 per annum gross, would be considered a high professional salary, and most families would have salaries between £550 and £1,100 per annum. The university generously pays £50 per annum for each child, but income tax takes back half of that.

Another general trend, in bringing up children, is towards a diminution in authoritarianism and an increase in permissiveness. With all new-found knowledge there is a great tendency to follow early exponents: and one of the earliest exponents, who advocated a very strict regime of child-rearing practice, was Truby King. He was the great pioneer in this country and yet recent inquiry showed that no librarian in Leeds had ever heard his name. Of course, this does not mean that feeding on demand has replaced feeding by time schedule. There are still doctors, nurses, health visitors, and textbooks which advocate a very rigid schedule of three-hourly feeds, followed at a later date by four-hourly feeds, but, especially among mothers who are not over-awed by their advisers, a relaxation of the rules often takes place.

A passage from a newly-published textbook for health visitors (23) shows that permissiveness can occur in the midst of orthodox and apparently rigid routine; 'When breast-feeding has been carried out regularly at three-hourly intervals from birth, the infant will automatically put itself on to four-hourly feeding when lactation is satisfactorily established. . . . This will happen about the sixth week but it may not be until the end of the third month.' Health visitors have told me that it is their regular practice to advise mothers to watch their child's need, and to reassure her that he will make his own schedule and that he knows what is best. Now this is a new doctrine coming in: that the baby knows best, not the expert. One health visitor, answering the question 'Do you advise that a baby should be fed when it cries, or at fixed intervals?' wrote 'A baby should be fed at fixed intervals but we usually find that he is fed at any time.'

Despite the strictness which the hospital tries to impose, only one mother of the university group fed by the clock and that was in the case of her first child; by the time her fourth and fifth children came along she was feeding completely on demand. This is an example of a cultural change taking place in one woman.

Opinion in Britain, both medical and lay, is unanimous that breast-feeding is best. It would be interesting to compare the time interval in Leeds between the birth and the time when the child is first put to the breast, with the same time lapse in New Guinea.[1] In Leeds it varies between 5 and 14 hours after birth, with an average of 9–10 hours. All the mothers questioned said they enjoyed breast-feeding.

Weaning takes place at from 5 to 10 months and is gradual; a comforter is not advised and very few are used nowadays. Usually between 5 and 6 months, solids are introduced gradually into the diet. At from 13 to 18 months the baby is feeding itself entirely by spoon. A baby who is partly weaned but continues the bottle is very unusual. I think the mothers feel that, having given the baby the breast up to about 8 or 9 months, he has had plenty and can just do without it.

With regard to toilet-training, there is a subtle but very marked difference from the attitude towards feeding. Perhaps this difference centres around the ingrained shame, secrecy and disgust which attaches to elimination, especially from the bowel. Prior to the mid-nineteenth century, families were sufficiently used to smells and untroubled by hygiene not to bother about training their children until control came naturally. The attitude to bowel-training in our time and generation is illustrated in the answers given by the university group of mothers to a question about playing with excrement: only three of the university mothers had ever noticed this in their children: one got very annoyed indeed and the other two 'removed the child swiftly'. But a health visitor said, in reply to the same question, 'Most young children will play with their faeces as they have no disgust. I advise mothers to say "Dirty" and to watch the child better in the future, and point out that this is quite natural in the child.' Now I am not sure whether the implication is that the sooner the baby gets over being natural the better, but it is noticeable how she swings from one opinion to another; she has read the books, but

[1] See p. 172.

her own innate disgust comes through, all the same. Another health visitor, on the other hand, had a more permissive attitude. She bemoaned the fact that very few mothers bothered to train the baby at all, but equally sadly she said of enuresis 'Mothers get far too cross, and this makes the baby feel guilty and ashamed. Often mother compares him with other children, to his detriment, and she ends by giving him a sound smacking.' About playing with faeces she said 'I advise the mother not to leave the child on the pot too long and not to scold, but to look on it as curiosity on his part and to accept it.'

In a film[1] that we made, there are two shots of potting. The first takes place in a day-nursery where infants are left while the mother is at work. A child is shown sitting on the pot on the nursery nurse's knee after a meal, crying in a resentful and yet a hopeless way, which reminded me of one of the children in Dr. Spitz's film *Grief*.[2] The cameraman was quite shocked with the barbaric scene of a room full of babies parked on their pots and rending the air with cries, but his professional interest made him say 'If only we were making a sound film, for no silent film can do justice to this scene!'

In another part of the film a child is seen refusing the pot in a vigorous and even athletic manner, while the mother wears a complex expression of distress on her face. It is not difficult to imagine what effect this behaviour may have upon the relationship between this mother and this child. These two scenes appear quite by chance; we did not set out to film antagonistic reactions to toilet-training, but rather attempted to show a sample of toilet-training, first as carried out in a group, and second in an individual home. Those in charge of the day-nursery saw and heard nothing unusual in what we filmed, for to them it was merely part of the daily routine. They were making no attempt to alter or improve the routine, for they saw nothing wrong or unusual in it.

When the individual mother agreed that we might film her child being potted, she said that he might not co-operate well and that she 'could not guarantee success'. So far as I know she has not consulted anyone because she does not consider her child's behaviour sufficiently abnormal. I cannot tell you what percentage of British children show distress or antagonism in their reaction to toilet-training, because information can only be obtained fortuitously. It is interesting that the textbook for health visitors, which contains 551 pages, devotes less than one page to toilet-training, and most of it is about micturition only.

Similarly, *Health of the Mother and Child* (8), published by the

---

[1] *Life Begins in Leeds*, see p. 222.
[2] See p. 103.

Department of Health for Scotland with the co-operation of the City of Glasgow, and distributed by the Central Council for Health Education, a booklet containing 66 pages of simple advice to mothers, devotes only ten lines to bowel-training and only seven to bladder control. There are, however, six lines on 'Bad Habits', which read 'Many normal children pass through a short stage of bad habits, but sometimes in spite of care and good upbringing bad habits may persist or a child may become backward, nervous and difficult. Very often this may have a bodily cause and in any case a doctor should be consulted, as a great deal can be done to restore normal development.' I do not think any politician could have done better! Here the section on bad habits ends, and whether the bad habits have to do with sex or toilet-training or just plain cussedness, this publication does not disclose. It gives a very nice picture of our attitude to these things.

Almost without exception the mothers in our inquiry had been advised to pot the child regularly before and after feeds, beginning soon after birth. It is very rare, they were told, for infants so trained to soil napkins after 3 months of age. This is perhaps not as extreme an assertion as one made by a famous Irish obstetrician in my hearing about a quarter of a century ago: he banged the desk quite angrily and said 'Every child should be trained in three weeks. All my children were trained in that way, and there is no need for any of this business about nappies and so on.'

Among the university mothers the tendency was to start toilet-training early, eleven out of fifteen children being potted regularly before they were a month old; one at 6 months, one at 8 months, one at 10 months, and one not until 20 months. Potting after the feed was the usual routine. Six mothers gave their children mild praise for good performance; two mothers expressed disapproval of wetting and soiling and called the child 'dirty' when he had made a mess; three mothers only, made some attempt to get the child to eliminate promptly, say within 10 minutes, and the others did not seem to mind. Only one mother encouraged reticence about elimination, and she 'always talked about it in a whisper'; the others either did not mind or their children were considered too young to be spoken to.

These several trends in child care and training seem to show, year by year, variations and alterations: they are surprisingly sensitive to various influences. Let no one think, for example, that their own influence in this field is unimportant, no matter what their job may be. Let no one think that their influence is likely to be lost in the total picture. Nor should it be supposed, in my opinion, that the Chichester Seminar can fail to have an influence upon these sensitive and ever-changing patterns. In Britain we have only to look back upon the effect of the Inter-departmental Committee on Physical Variation in 1904, or the first National Conference on Infant Mortality, in 1906, to see that the effect was to turn the tide which had run strongly in favour of artificial feeding from the latter half of the eighteenth century, to run strongly in favour of breast-feeding. In other words, if a conference can make up its mind really firmly even about one thing, it may have a vast effect. It is true that it may have to deal with matters more complicated and subtle than the simple choice between breast- and bottle-feeding, but, on the other hand, an examination of the motives which lie behind the choice shows that they bear a marked resemblance to those influences which determine the total emotional attitude of the mother to her child. A change such as this will not be just nation-wide; it will be part of an almost universal ironing-out of cultural and local customs, a world-wide process of levelling of the social strata.

THE UNITED KINGDOM
CASE HISTORIES[1]

D. R. MacCalman

THE CASE MATERIAL from the United Kingdom, as befits our island, is small in quantity. The abnormal cases were selected from children referred to our Child Guidance Clinic in Leeds, and we chose those who were as young as possible and whose mothers appeared to be interested and co-operative. More dramatic material and a wider choice would have been possible if we had extended our age range, but we felt that the memories of mothers for detailed information are quite short, and that it might not reach far enough back to give us the kind of material we wanted. Another reason for the small quantity of material is that the Department of Psychological Medicine in the University of Leeds is quite young, and it is only in the last three years that we have been able to do any appreciable amount of children's work. The Department itself was only instituted in 1946 and before that the region was very backward in psychiatric work. Prior to the National Health Service there were large, over-crowded mental hospitals with very small medical staffs, and the first job was to improve these hospitals, by securing proper staffing, and by establishing out-patient departments in the various cities and districts of the region.

There was a great deal to do before introducing 'refinements', as child guidance is regarded in Yorkshire, not only by the public, but also by the medical profession, the education authorities and the schools. It was no easy task to introduce the idea that families can be helped in the bringing up of their children. That was traditionally left to parents, who were supposed to handle their own children without any outside help. There are many proverbs which indicate that family troubles must be kept within the household.

It is noteworthy that in the Peter R. case[1] we had no contact with the father at all, and when the mother was asked whether the father would come to the clinic, she immediately became anxious and asked whether he would be told what she had been saying. She explained that he was antagonistic to the idea of Peter attending the clinic as he felt that there was a strong stigma attached to such attendance.

[1] See Vol. II, Part III.

71

Mrs. R. herself said that she would be only too pleased if her husband would attend, provided the staff would not discuss with him any family differences he might bring up. She felt so strongly about it that even a home visit would have been injudicious.

In a psychiatric service in an area where there is a stigma attached to psychiatric work, the best propaganda is efficient help, that is, successful treatment of cases. The clinic, in fact, has to play the good father and good mother role to ensure any success.

A second principle has been put into words by Dr. Bowlby, that there should be no research without therapy, and no therapy without research. Further, we were anxious, in the Peter R. case, not to spoil our relationship with the paediatrician. There is, of course, quite a feeling between paediatricians and child psychiatrists in this country, to some extent because the paediatrician, with noted exceptions, does not really believe that the psychiatrist can treat children more efficiently than he can.

Again, we did not want to upset our link with the school and the education department because this is also delicate ground. The teachers feel that they know their own business and want nobody coming in to tell them how to handle their problem children. We had also to keep in mind the friends and relatives in the area, because news travels round very quickly and negative feelings are soon translated into gossip. And while there is considerable delicacy about cases in which help has been sought, there is even more delicacy in cases where no advance is made at all, as in the 'normal' cases we studied.

These 'normal' cases were obtained indirectly through such bodies as the local education authorities, psychologists, or voluntary religious societies. We felt that a favour was being sought, because these mothers were busy women who had no domestic help; their time was valuable and their leisure practically non-existent. We were also causing them a certain amount of embarrassment by some of the questions we asked. Any suggestion that the child should be tested or interviewed alone, or examined medically or psychiatrically, might easily have spoiled the contact with the case.

One mother who was contacted laid down certain conditions before she would say anything at all. These conditions were as follows: 1. That the psychiatrist should never have anything to do with her child; 2. That no attempt should be made to see the child, even indirectly at the school, by anyone whatsoever; 3. That no attempt should be made to persuade the parents to come to the department at any time or on any pretext. Finally, the child's father said that he did not want to have anything to do with the plan because he did not think the child should have any contact with mentally defective children! You can see that the investigator could do nothing but terminate the interview as gracefully as possible. That is the kind of community in which we work and the reason why we have to tread delicately. The anxiety about mentally defective children is not surprising, because for many years there has been a well-developed and active department of the local authority, called, euphemistically, the mental health department, concerned with the community care and training of the dull and backward, and the mentally defective children and adults. This mother was not to be blamed for correlating in her mind the problem of intellectual retardation and the stigma attached to another organization dealing with other aspects of mental health.

The 'normal' cases are, therefore, little more than impressionistic studies; worth putting in because they give some contrast to the abnormal cases. As far as possible these cases were balanced against the abnormal cases in family structure, in age, in intelligence, and in socio-economic background.

Of the first pair of children studied,[1] Charles was an only child and so was Andrew, both 5-plus in age, both highly intelligent, although with regard to Andrew we can only judge by his performance at school. They both lived in 'pre-fab' houses on a housing estate. The other two children[2] were Jewish, both were under 5, both of average intelligence, both came from middle-class families, and, interestingly enough, the span between the parents' marriage and the birth of the child was long in both cases: six years in the case of Peter and ten and a half years in that of Michael.

Of the four British cases, only the mother of Andrew was able to enjoy her child for what he was, and to accept him as he was. The others were anxious to change their children in some way, and could take no serene happiness in them.

In the questionnaire used in our inquiries, we put in a section on games, songs and pastimes—because the degree to which a family is rich in that kind of material shows the depth of its original background, and is quite a good measure of family stability; although it may also indicate the degree to which the family is living in the past, unable to make progress into the future. Our questionnaire was given orally to all except the university mothers, who answered it in writing by themselves. It began with a section dealing with health. That is a good way of starting with people whom one does not know, for fathers and mothers will always talk about the health of their children quite easily and openly. No advice was given to the mothers of normal children, but any quite obvious help was given to them, and some of their needs met.

[1] Cases studied at the Seminar, but not included in Vol. II.   [2] See Vol. II, Part III.

It seems worth while to comment on the fact that the topics of punishment and discipline were at no time prominent in the discussions at Chichester. Discipline and control are, of course, implicit in the difference between the flexible and rigid schedules. What explanation can there be for this apparent lack of interest in the matter of punishment? Prof. Meredith suggested that it might be because there were not many teachers present at the Seminar, and that in infancy the situation scarcely arises. Babies in cots do not give as much trouble as they are apt to do later.

I am inclined to think that we in the United Kingdom are more preoccupied with discipline than the French or Americans. Can this pre-occupation be related to our history, which is particularly rich in reactions to authority, from the days of Magna Carta onwards? The feudal system must have given rise to marked ambivalence between serfs and over-lords, and there was an interesting difference between the feudal system and the clan system in Scotland. The latter involved the government by, and the allegiance of people of the same name to, a hereditary chief. This kinship system had this important difference from the feudal system, that there was no compulsion on the individual to follow his chief. He could join a neighbouring clan if he thought the conditions of service were better there. Perhaps this lack of compulsion explains the failure of the last attempt of the Stuart royal line to regain the throne in 1745. Bonnie Prince Charlie, Charles Edward Stuart, the Young Pretender, swept all before him in his advance from Scotland until he came to Derby. London was wide open, but the clans were tired of the campaign and they exercised their right to return with their booty to their wives and families. This may be another example of the family being fundamentally asocial, so far as the wider affairs of the community or nation are concerned. This was certainly true in the 1939–45 war, when separation anxiety accounted for more breakdowns than battle experiences, even among ammunition workers merely asked to go from London to Lancashire. The breakdown rate among the Civil Servants who went in a body from Whitehall to places like Bournemouth was extremely high; those who broke down could not apparently bear to be even that short distance away from their accustomed zone of bureaucracy.

The industrial revolution gave rise to another example of conflict, but the effects of that conflict were minimized by the Puritan tradition, which approved of poverty because the only true reward would come, not on this earth, but in Heaven. In fact, the whole doctrine of Puritanism might have been written by a propagandist employed by the early industrialists! The discomforts of life, the fruits of poverty, were jewels in the crown of the martyrs. The hard way was good in itself, and as Shakespeare said 'The primrose path leads but to the grave'.

An important factor in family tradition in Britain is that the Bible, and in particular the Old Testament, used to be read in so many households at morning prayers every day. Quotations from the Bible came readily to the lips of our ancestors, and play a part in the authoritarian aspects of our traditions. Quotations like 'Spare the rod and spoil the child', 'Honour thy father and thy mother', gave sanction to rigid schedules.

These sentiments have an archaic ring, but they have played a fundamentally important part in the personality structure of the mothers and grandmothers of our patients, on whom they and their children were so dependent for their stability and adjustment, or the reverse. One point comes out of the study of case material from all the countries: that the greatest good fortune one can have is a stable and well-doing family background.

One group at Chichester discussed the fact that we talk in Britain not of a thrashing or a beating but of a *good* thrashing or a *sound* beating; there was also the favourite threat in my own childhood of, 'Your bottom will be well warmed'. In contrast, some of the Latin races utter violent threats to a child, but in an endearing and caressing tone of voice. A mother may scream delightedly, 'I shall kill you', or a father might say to his son, 'I'll tear your liver out'. The group noted too the importance of the parent having a certain natural compassion for the child in trouble. Parents must be able to tolerate their own hatred of the child at certain times, but the difficulty which the British mother has in tolerating this spontaneous and natural hatred is very considerable.

Against such a background the amount and kind of punishment which characterizes, for example, Scottish education, is neither as surprising nor as traumatic to those punished as might appear to one not so reared. You can imagine the upset, the chaos even, which followed the publications of A. S. Neill, who himself was the son of an Aberdeenshire schoolmaster. I remember well the delight with which he received the small son of an Aberdeenshire farmer whom I recommended to him in 1935. This was the first child from his native county who had ever been sent to his school. Some of his books are historical documents: *The Dominie's Log, A Dominie Dismissed, Problem Parents, Problem Teachers,* and *Problem Children.* He advocated freedom of sex education and this, of course, was partly responsible for the reputation he gained of being a heretic.

The experiences of Neill's and Bertrand Russell's schools in England did a great deal to undermine the authority of the parents, or rather, to sap the confidence which parents formerly had in their authority. They had felt it was their duty to punish for the child's good. In some cases there has been a swing from rigid discipline to the opposite extreme. This has produced a great deal of parental anxiety and accounts for many of the insecure, obsessional, and hostile children whom we are used to seeing at the clinics.

A mother and daughter illustrated this anxiety quite markedly. When the two of them came to the clinic it was impossible to separate them, and I could see why. This small child of 4 and her mother sat there watching each other like fighting cocks, with great hostility towards each other. It looked as if it would be a pretty even battle with just a hint of superiority on the side of the child. At last we managed to separate them and I had the child to myself. In a pause in the conversation, I asked her what she would like to do when she grew up. Her answer came quite promptly, as follows: 'I shall get married when I grow up and I shall have children and I shall be very good to them and love them a lot until they are 3 years old and then I shall pitch them out of the window.'

The story behind this was that the mother was one of a family of five girls, amongst whom there was a good deal of rivalry as to who should get married first. They all married before this girl, who was rather plainer than the others and perhaps more inhibited. Before she married she would visit her sisters and their families and no doubt she had some jealous feeling. She was critical of her nephews and nieces, mainly because she thought they were uncontrolled and undisciplined. The sisters would laugh and say, 'Wait until you have a child and then we will see who is spoiled.' When she became pregnant, she was determined that she would not spoil her child as her sisters did theirs, but when the baby was born it seemed so small and helpless that, persuading herself that discipline did not matter to begin with, she poured out all her love on the child. She went so far that, when the child was three years old, and there was a family gathering, her sisters rocked with laughter because the child was so spoiled. Horrified and angry with herself, she completely changed her attitude towards her child and became rigid in her discipline and severe in her punishments.

There was a time in our history, chiefly in the 'thirties', when parents were confused: tradition bade them to punish and be severe, but the current fashion was to give complete freedom. Gradually this confusion has died away, and not only in Britain, for now we can have an international Seminar without getting too anxious about control and discipline.

DISCUSSION

In discussion it was stated that health services in Britain do a surprising amount for the people, but in many cases families do not attempt to get help, even of the most simple kind. This is a measure of their independence, of their feeling that it is letting the family down to seek help in any way.

Very often the psychiatrist is thought to be a charlatan by a physician who feels completely discouraged in the face of a case which has nothing to do with general medicine; on the other hand, a person can attend a hospital for many years with a succession of complaints before it occurs to anybody that there may be a psychiatric aspect, and then they confidently expect the psychiatrist to produce a miracle. Many physicians think of psychiatric disorders, neurotic and delinquent behaviour, as based on some conscious determination on the part of the individual, as though one only had to point out the error of their ways and people would be changed from being obsessional or hallucinated or whatever it might be; but there is considerable difficulty, if not complete impossibility, in treating, say, a woman of 55 who has been obsessional all her life.

Questions regarded as intimate are not always about sex. In some countries there are many more compromising questions, including perhaps a question as to the person's political views. In America a child will not talk about whether he has enough to eat. He might say that his father beat his mother, or his father got drunk, but to the question, 'Do you get enough to eat?' he would not be able to bear to say that his parents could not give him enough to eat; that would be the *intimate* question.

POPULAR MAGAZINES AND THE UPBRINGING OF CHILDREN

Fernando Henriques

OVER A PERIOD of about a year, Mrs. Mestel, of the University of Leeds Department of Psychology, collected material dealing with child rearing out of a number of popular magazines.

This material would be difficult to understand without considerable background knowledge about Great Britain. Dr. Aubry (Dr. Jenny Roudinesco) emphasized that France is composed of regions of varying character, and this also applies to the United States and, I think, to Great Britain, for underneath the superficial structure and political unity of the British Isles there is an enormous variation. The first factor of differentiation is the locale, or situation; and another is employment. Then there is a difference in housing, traditions, customs, folklore; all, to a large extent, govern the way in which people live. We are apt to conclude that because people live in a highly industrialized area, such things as traditions and folklore disappear. In a working-class district in Britain there is as much magic as in any country in Europe; a different kind of magic, but basically the same.

Factors of unity can also be described. What really unites the country as a political and social unity? There is a common loyalty to a political creed, again with a great number of local variations, but basically the same. There are the major institutions, such as the family and marriage, the law, and so on, which are common to the whole country. Radio and popular literature are only comparatively recent developments; but despite the factors of differentiation there is a form of unity in the popular magazine, which makes for a sort of stereotyped response of people to this type of communication stimulus.

There is one point of contrast between the U.K. and France which, I think, is quite fundamental. In France the urban worker never really loses his contact with the land; he may have relatives still living on the land though he himself is working in a city; his children are sent from the city to spend weeks or months with the grandmother in the country. But whereas over 50 per cent of the people in France gain their living from agriculture, in the U.K. the figure is as low as 15 per cent; and this means that the community

78

is of a different type. The reason for this is that this country was the first in the world to become industrialized, and thus early destroyed its rural and peasant heritage.

In examining these magazines against the background of a highly structured society, we have divided them into groups which correspond to the class-structure of society. Group I, for instance, represents the middle-to-upper-class section of society; Group II, the middle-to-lower-middle-classes, and Group III the working-class or lower classes. Such a grouping is only possible because, as a result of compulsory education, most people can read.

One or other of the Group III magazines goes into every working-class home in the country, and no other form of literature is read by these people. The men read the sporting and racing papers, and the football pools—a recent major phenomenon. People spend a great deal of their week-ends in making football pool forecasts. Some people do well at it; others have been filling in coupons for fifteen years without winning a penny, but the disease has spread widely in Europe and the British Dominions and is a phenomenon which might possibly change the structure of social life.

In grouping the magazines into three categories, no single criterion has been used. Price seems to have very little to do with it. *Family Doctor* in Group I, published by the British Medical Association, costs 1s. 6d.; while *True Story Magazine* in Group III costs 1s. 3d. The criteria are: the quality of the fiction, the stylishness of the fashion pages, the imaginativeness of the recipes, and the presence or absence of astrological guides. Two hundred and seventy-five magazine issues were surveyed and were selected for study because of their psychological importance, and because some of them are the subject of disagreement among the experts.

The table shows, graphically, the topics which have been treated and the relative amount of attention given them. For example, in Group I, there were three times as many articles concerned with feeding as with pregnancy, children's ailments, sleeping problems, and so on. There are many interesting observations to be made.

Childbirth. A great deal of attention is paid, especially in Group III, to the problems of pregnancy and childbirth. Dr. Grantly Dick Read's views on natural childbirth, ante-natal exercises and especially relaxation, are recommended by fourteen magazines, from the lowest grade (*Lucky Star* and *Peg's Paper*), to first-class magazines like *Good Housekeeping*. There was no criticism of relaxation or natural childbirth in any magazine.

Infant Feeding. Another favourite topic is feeding—breast- or bottle-feeding. The virtues of breast-feeding are emphasized by ten magazines,

PROPORTION OF SUCH TOPICS DISCUSSED

	GROUP I 5 magazines 30 issues	GROUP II 5 magazines 50 issues	GROUP III 5 magazines 50 issues
PROBLEM OR TOPIC			
problems of conception and its social aspects			
pregnancy and confinement			
feeding			
elimination			
prevention and cure of illness			
teething			
motor development			
safety			
sleep and its problems			
clothing (excluding patterns)			
bathing and cleanliness			
perambulators and other equipment			
outings, travelling			
fresh air and sunshine			
games, songs stories and toys			
speech			
discipline			
temper tantrums			
separation of parents and child			
role of father			
conflict with other adults over upbringing			
relations with older brothers and sisters			
problems of mentally defective children			

The attention given to different aspects of child-rearing in fifteen popular magazines.

at all levels; and of these, eight give advice on the preparation of the breasts and on methods of increasing a dwindling milk supply. A further six also implicitly support breast-feeding. Where the advantages of breast-feeding are listed, four out of nine magazines confine themselves to the physical advantages, five include some reference to the psychological importance, one mentions the emotional satisfaction given to the mother. No magazine recommends bottle-feeding if breast-feeding is at all possible. The general attitude expressed towards bottle-feeding is, 'What a pity it is necessary, but don't worry, we will help you to make the best of it.'

Feeding Schedule. Only one magazine (Group III), in discussing the relative merits of schedule and 'self-demand' feeding, definitely comes down on the side of the former, on the grounds that the baby would in any case make a four-hourly schedule for himself. In no case is a really strict schedule on Truby King lines recommended.

In five magazines (two in Group III and three in Group II) which assume the existence of the conventional four-hourly schedule, some slackening is recommended; for example, allowing night-feeding and permitting as much as an hour's latitude for the 6 a.m. and 10 p.m. feeds. Three magazines (all Group I) advocate 'self-demand' feeding.

Solid Food. All magazines give between 4 and 5 months, and when the weight is from 14 to 15 lbs., as the time when solids should be introduced into the baby's diet. In one magazine there was an article describing children who had been given a completely liquid diet of milk and honey until 2 years of age, but an editorial comment discouraged other mothers from carrying out this regime. Six magazines, evenly distributed among the groups, varied in their ideal time to begin weaning, from six months, spread over ten weeks, to nine months, spread over five weeks. Two magazines mentioned that 'it would do no harm' to breast-feed until 1 year. In all cases weaning should be gradual, taking five to ten weeks, and dropping one breast-feed after the other. Two magazines advocate nine months' breast-feeding, but realize that few mothers can manage so long 'under modern conditions'. Two magazines in Group III point out that it is not necessary to wean because menstruation has begun during nursing.

Thumb-Sucking. Thumb-sucking is condemned by two magazines as the cause of wind and a deformer of teeth. It should not, however, be prevented forcibly, but ignored, and attention given to the child's emotional satisfaction. Dummies are condemned for the same reasons. One Group III and one Group I magazine positively recommend the use of dummies, either as preferable to thumb-sucking, or as a justifiable comfort to an unhappy child.

Feeding Problems. Refusal to eat receives attention in six magazines (three in Group I, one in Group II, one in Groups II and III, and one in Group III) which advise mothers 'Don't be anxious, don't force food, and don't let the child become the centre of attention.' One magazine in Group II recommends getting at the root of the matter, which may be jealousy or unhappiness of some sort, and putting it

G 81

right. One, in Group III, in its answer to a problem of a girl of 12 months who holds the food in her mouth and then spits it out, advises what it considers to be a better chosen diet.

Four magazines tell the mother to encourage her child to feed himself. Three of them advise her not to worry if he makes a mess, and to let him feed himself with his fingers if he wants to. On the other hand, one magazine advises a mother to continue spoon-feeding her 20-months old son, who is still more interested in playing with his food and the utensils than in eating.

Toilet-Training. Three magazines advise potting the baby from the start. One writes: 'We would like to teach Reginald Robert his manners, too, while he is with us (at the hospital). We shall introduce him to the pottie to-morrow (the day after his birth) for we want his baby mind to connect up the pottie with what he is supposed to do in it.' The other two make the proviso that it should be taken gently and not too much expected of the child. One, in Group II, discusses in some detail whether to begin training early or late, and decides for early training on the grounds that the late introduction of the pot will leave the child bewildered and confused, and will release hostile feelings which will be expressed in every aspect of his life.

One magazine in Group I recommends leaving toilet-training until the child is old enough to understand what is expected of him. Nine magazines deal with the various problems of toilet-training—mainly the angry refusal of the pot by a recalcitrant child and the mother's subsequent despair. Their advice is unanimous: 'Don't worry, don't expect too much, never battle over the pot, nor scold for failures.'

Sleep Difficulties. Reluctance to go to sleep, and night-crying, receive a good deal of attention. The idea of 'being firm and letting them cry it out' when all physical needs have been satisfied is condemned by four magazines. The three Group I magazines recommend such solutions as a happy bed-time ritual, staying with the child until he goes to sleep, sleeping in the same room as a temporary measure, giving reassurance, affection and comfort, as well as the usual physical aids (alterations in diet, more exercise, and so on). 'Letting them cry it out' is advocated by three magazines, all in Group III, on the grounds that the child will become spoilt and 'try it on' if he is pandered to. Two magazines say that a certain amount of crying is natural and healthy, and can therefore be ignored.

Discipline. Those magazines which discuss the general basis of discipline are all concerned to relax the strict attitude which they say many parents have towards their children. Three magazines tell mothers to expect naughtiness and sometimes even unpleasant behaviour, but warn them against taking it too tragically. One magazine points out that children have no sense of right or wrong at this age, that the need for firmness is not so great as some mothers suppose. On the other hand, there should be calm assurance and, above all, consistency. Mothers are recommended to act skilfully and cut down the occasions for bad behaviour, and to offer attractive substitutes for forbidden things. Angry smacks are definitely condemned by two Group II magazines. Three magazines say that parents must agree about, and share responsibility for, discipline.

Temper Tantrums. In five magazines the advice, on the whole, is to treat temper tantrums as a common occurrence, and to try to understand the motives and show the child sympathy and understanding. The child should be made to feel he is loved and that he is capable of doing things. A wise mother will try to prevent the tantrums. Two magazines assure mothers that the terrifying practice of breath-holding is not to be worried about, and one recommends the application of a cold sponge.

Jealousy. Four magazines deal with, for example, the problem of telling the older child when a new baby is due. With children up to 6 years, it is advisable to treat the matter naturally and only tell the child as much as he asks for. Suggestions made include acting the new birth with the older child's dolls, showing the older child babies in prams, and avoiding the impression that the new baby can be in any way a playmate. One magazine recommends not telling a child of 6 years until six weeks before the confinement, 'as children's memories are so short'. Two Group II magazines state that it is better for the older child to stay in his familiar surroundings, with someone he knows, during the confinement.

Sibling jealousy between brothers and sisters is touched on by nine magazines. One advises giving the older child plenty of responsibility and making him feel grown up. Sympathy and extra affection for the older child are advised by seven, while four go so far as to warn the mother against neglecting the baby in her efforts not to make the older child feel pushed out. One advises discussing the question with the child. Two magazines say that if the older child wishes, he should be allowed to use a bottle, revert to nappies, and so on.

The Father's Role. Apart from mentioning the importance of both parents sharing discipline, scarcely any magazines deal with the father's role. One, in Group II, advises the 'father-to-be' on how to treat his wife during her pregnancy. Another, in Group III, says that a wife who does not go out to work should not expect, as a matter of course, any help from her husband with the early morning feed, and should be grateful for any she receives, because the husband must have an undisturbed night's sleep, since the wife can always make it up during the day. Father can help at week-ends. Another Group III magazine suggests that father's playing with his 18 months old daughter in the evening is making her over-excited, and should be limited to the week-ends.

Separation. Two magazines definitely advise that the mother of a young child should not go out to work if it can be avoided. Two Group I magazines give a full-length feature on the W.H.O. Technical Report on Maternal Care and Mental Health (Bowlby) (2) with full approval of its conclusions, although one of these, on another occasion, included an article by a day-nursery matron approving day-nurseries wholeheartedly, without any reservation as to the child's age. One other magazine says that no child should go to a day-nursery before 2 years, and very few at that age.

Literary Quality. The literary quality declines from Group I to Group III. In Group III, the most productive because of its variety, one magazine has a feature entitled 'The Family Doctor' with a little picture of a doctor seated at his desk, looking very benevolent, bursting to answer questions.

The stories in the magazines have exciting titles, they begin in a dramatic manner, and the endings are perfectly moral. It seems a little strange that this type of literature should be so extraordinarily popular in the highly sophisticated society in which we live.

DISCUSSION

An interesting point in connection with the magazines under discussion is the rate at which they are read. During a twelve-hour train journey a young soldier was seen to start on the first page of a comic paper and go through it methodically; on arrival he was half way down page 4. It is the same with the popular press. The standard of literacy in the U.K. is open to question: many people 'read' the comics merely by looking at the pictures.

The question is, what should be done about these magazines? Should professional people volunteer to run columns in the magazines, and if so, would they do any better than is already done?

Readers Digest, which has a very wide circulation, has, in each number, a medical article of a high order. During the last two years articles have appeared about children, child care and maternity; natural childbirth has been discussed and a good deal written about experiments in solving family difficulties, adoption, breast-feeding, and the significance of the psychological reaction between mother and child.

Since World War II, magazines in the U.S.A. have devoted more and more space to discussion of medical issues and problems. In 1947 the *Saturday Evening Post*, for the first time in its history, had a medical article—on epilepsy in children; most magazines since, of all classes, have carried articles on medical problems more or less regularly. It has made general practitioners feel that the public is getting too well-educated in relation to general medical problems, and a need arises for the general practitioner to educate himself further about what illness means to the whole family, and not only to the person who is ill; as, for example, the effects on the rest of the family, and the adjustments they have to make.

The experience of the Paediatric Department at the University of Sydney, Australia, with regard to matters such as tuberculosis and rheumatic fever, and certain aspects of endocrinology, which have a popular appeal, is to have been bombarded by the Press for statements. Subjects like the possible part endocrines play in pregnancy and the formation of the infant, appeal greatly to the Press.

In the U.K. the *Family Doctor* is published by the British Medical Association in an attempt to provide an attractive magazine to counteract some of the influence of other magazines.

There is a common danger that better educated people will feel above writing in the Class III magazines.

Harper's Magazine, a Class I magazine, wanted Dr. Margaret Mead to re-write a chapter from *Male and Female* for them to publish, considering that the book itself was too difficult for many of their readers. After re-writing, the editors still felt it was too difficult. However, *Ladies Home Journal*, more of Class II level, published a quarter of the book in the original vocabulary, and experienced no difficulty whatever. They did not despise their readers, who, they believed, could use a dictionary to look up a word which they did not understand.

This contempt is one of the big problems in the relationship between the popular press and the learned professions; it is often shared by the editors of magazines.

How can one deal directly with the Press? In New York, the National Association for Mental Health employs an officer to work with the Press, and, furnished with the best advice, he can re-write and arrange material for the Press so well that the publishers come to prefer to get it from him.

Who writes the articles—qualified persons, doctors, nurses or lay journalists? In many cases it is not possible to find out. The *Family*

Doctor has all the best experts, as has the *Nursery World*; in Group II and Group III magazines, the part played by matrons and nurses is very large.

There was only one reference to sex education in the magazines, and occasionally something about telling children 'where babies come from'.

In France this type of literature is rather different, and more often than not women's journals are concerned with troubles of the heart. Unhappy women write about their problems, and perhaps a professor of psychiatry would not be the best authority to answer them. Usually, the answers are very prudent and moral.

On a more general point, although in the industrial areas of Great Britain the rural or peasant heritage has largely disappeared, the Agricultural Workers' Union is still the largest of the single craft unions, and the rural heritage is still strong in rural parts of the country.

United States of America

CHILD DEVELOPMENT PATTERNS IN THE UNITED STATES

Edith B. Jackson

DR. ETHELYN H. KLATSKIN, my associate at Yale, suggested that the essential idea with which to introduce this subject should be the impossibility of any discussion, except theoretical, of any average development in the United States, for three reasons. The first was the variation over the country as a whole, with its many differences in climate and population groups. For instance, it has been suggested that in the south-west, relatively less clothing and less bundling up in the winter, and greater space for family living, may be conducive to earlier gross motor development, with earlier standing and walking.

The second reason was the range of variation within any given aspect of development. There are various aspects of development of which the psychologist speaks: e.g., gross and fine motor development (of large and small muscles), speech development (language response), adaptive response (to inanimate objects) and social-personal response (to people).

The third reason was the evidence that the norms are in process of changing.

Dr. Sally Provence of the Yale Child Study Centre also mentioned the variability and the lack of definitely predictable patterns of behaviour for the United States child. She outlined three quite different developmental 'profiles' of behaviour at the ages of 3, 6, 9 and 12 months of three normal healthy infants, all receiving good care from normal healthy mothers. The profiles appeared to demonstrate the importance not only of individual constitutional factors, but also of the interaction of these with extrinsic or environmental factors. Although, at present, most observers agree only that in a group of infants definite inborn differences are discernible from the neo-natal period onwards, it is possible that the accumulation of many detailed studies of behaviour profiles may lead to the recognition of various general types of normal infant development.

There is evidence that growth and rate of development in the present generation of North American infants has significantly advanced over the norms established on the Gesell, Cattell and Viennese infant developmental scales. For instance, Dr. Klatskin has recently reported (15) on the development of 184 infants followed up in the Yale Rooming-in Project[1] as compared with Cattell's norms. The rooming-in infants showed a significantly higher percentage, in general about 10 per cent, of success on most items of the scale, with the constant exception of vocabulary.

A study by Howard V. Meredith in 1943 (19) revealed that the average 2-year-old infant was 4 cm. or $1\frac{1}{2}$ in. taller in 1940 than in 1880. The reduction of sickness and the improvement in health and nutrition through public health regulations and medical supervision have been notable during those years and are regarded as responsible for this change in the norm of growth. It does not appear that these shifts in the motor developmental rate are related to social and economic status.

Dr. Klatskin's report summarizes the possible influences as follows:

'Improved paediatric care has been suggested as partly responsible for such shifts. Peatman and Higgons (21) have shown that the average ages for sitting, standing, and walking in the group of children raised with optimal paediatric care are lower than the norms for these developmental stages as reported by Gesell and Thompson (11) for the same period. The report of Peatman and Higgons was based on children born before 1940 and apparently raised on fixed feeding regimes with less general self-regulation than is practised in the rooming-in group. It is interesting to note, therefore, that the percentage they report as walking at 52 weeks (44 per cent), though above the percentage reported by Gesell and Thompson (26 per cent), is below that of the present group (61 per cent). In addition, it seems probable that cultural changes toward less confining clothing for infants may permit more exercise in the early months of life . . . It is also plausible to assume that the amount of parental attention and handling, and consequent exercise and stimulation, received by a group of infants on self-regulated regimes is greater than that received by infants on strict schedules, as was customary during the period when Cattell's norms were established. The possibility of such an effect has been suggested by Trainham and by Gilliland (13).'

In presenting a general survey of the normal range of variation in the developmental pattern of United States infants, as at present understood by professional workers and conveyed to parents through professional contacts or through parent manuals, I have taken the

[1] In the Yale Rooming-in Project, mothers having their confinements in the University Hospital were allowed, if they wished, to have their babies with them, instead of in a special babies' nursery.

two most widely read manuals in the United States as guides: Spock's *Pocket Book of Baby and Child Care* published in 1946 (26), and the ninth edition of the Children's Bureau publication, *Infant Care*, published by the Federal Security Agency of the United States in 1951 (17). Of course, all parents do not read baby care literature; some are dependent for guidance on the older generation, or on doctors and nurses in welfare clinics. In any case whether they read or whether they just listen, they do not necessarily follow the suggested ways. The non-readers, at the present time, are apt to be more dependent on schedule and more restrictive, probably because of the influence of their more strictly brought-up parents.

American parents who avail themselves of the above-mentioned literature on infant care are immediately introduced to the fact of variation in the way babies grow and develop, not only as a matter of physical constitution but also a matter of their own response to the child. On the very first page of *Infant Care* this statement occurs: 'Something of what your baby is going to be was determined before he was born . . . Those who are around him in his first year will have a lot to do with whether or not he finds the world a good place, and is joyful and glad to be alive.' In the section on 'Development', sixty pages on, we read that each baby is different, that each baby sets his own pace, and that development follows a pattern. 'Instead of looking for a *time* when certain things will appear, look for the *order* in which to expect them.' Thus, an underlying order of human development is emphasized. Spock says his advice to parents to enjoy each child for what he is, is not given just for sentimental reasons. 'There is a very important practical point here. The child who is appreciated for what he is . . . will grow up with confidence in himself, happy . . . But the child who has never been quite accepted by his parents, who has always felt he was not quite right, grows up lacking confidence and is not able to make full use . . . of what capacities he has.' Spock also emphasizes the underlying order of behaviour in human development before discussing variations.

Among the variations the question of 'three-month colic' or irritable fussiness in the early months of life is discussed at length. In the U.S.A. what determines the difference between the many 'good babies' who thrive and develop with very little trouble from the beginning and the many babies who are fussy, fretful and 'colicky' in the early months of life is not satisfactorily understood.

According to our source books, it is normal for a baby to hold his head up when pulled to a sitting position at 2 to 4 months. He reaches out and grasps objects between 4 and 6 months. He laughs out loud at about 4 months, and notices and responds to people.

Shyness on seeing strange people or things may begin at 5 to 6 months, and is usually over by 1 year. This phenomenon has no clear explanation. One wonders whether it was present when the household unit was larger than it is to-day. It has been pointed out that such shyness is a sign that the child is now able to distinguish between mother and strangers.

The American child, according to *Infant Care*, sits up some time between 6 and 8 months. Crawling begins from 7 to 9 months, according to *Infant Care*, and from 6 to 12 months according to Spock. The suggestion is made to mothers that they should start using the play-pen before the child actually begins to crawl—this may be as early as 4, 5, or 6 months. The play-pen is used, in my experience, mostly from 6 to 10 months, and very seldom after a year.

The child usually pulls himself up to a standing position at 9 to 10 months. He takes a little while to learn to sit down again. The use of apparatus to assist in walking so that he can propel himself along is advised against, at least for more than a short period; but the child who is standing alone may, of course, walk alone very soon. This may happen by the end of the first year. According to Spock, 'Most babies learn to walk between 12 and 15 months. A few . . . start as early as 9 months, but a fair number, who are not suffering from any disease, do not begin until 18 months or even later.' That leaves a tremendous amount of leeway.

In Dr. Klatskin's investigations of the rooming-in children 66 per cent were walking at the end of 52 weeks. She was not able to find a control group to test whether children who were on a rigid schedule would show any difference in this development, because the idea of flexibility in the management of children was so diffused throughout the community that it made it impossible to find subjects for a control survey.

As for speech, there is very general agreement that the first words are apt to appear about the end of the first year. They may appear before or after the child has started to walk. Development of speech is not wholly dependent on muscular control. Speech learning, once begun, may be interrupted by a concentration on learning to do something else, generally walking, and it may be well in the second year or even later before the child begins to put words together. Variations seem to depend on temperament and personality and on the way the child is handled. *Infant Care* calls attention to the fact that the child can understand what is said to him and can sense the feeling of what is said about him even before he speaks. Therefore parents are cautioned to be careful and say only things which will make the baby feel comfortable.

Apparently, there is great need in the U.S.A. to caution parents not to be in too much of a hurry to know whether the child is left-handed or right-handed, and not to try to change him if it looks as if he were going to be left-handed. It may be difficult in the first year to tell which hand the child is going to use; handedness is sometimes not determined until the second or third years.

A smaller percentage of the mothers in the U.S.A. breast-feed than is reported for other countries. There are great variations in this regard in different sections of the country. For instance, according to Dr. Katherine Bain's figures in 1947 (1), in the south-eastern section 82 per cent are discharged from the hospital on breast or breast plus a supplementary formula. In the north-east section only 39 per cent are discharged on breast or breast plus bottle. In the State of Connecticut as a whole 30 per cent are discharged on breast, with or without formula. According to our own figures during the year 1947, 43 per cent were discharged from the New Haven Hospital on breast or breast plus bottle. 17 per cent of the rooming-in mothers who left the hospital nursing their babies continued to nurse for 6 months or longer. 10 per cent of the non-rooming-in mothers continued to nurse for 6 months or longer.

Solid foods are introduced early, usually at 3 or 4 months, although it may be even earlier, and occasionally later. Considerable latitude is allowed regarding the type of solids introduced. They may be either cereal or stewed fruit, at first, and vegetable puree and soups soon afterwards.

A good many babies want to begin to feed themselves before one year. Parents are urged to shut their eyes to the mess the child makes on beginning to feed himself and not to worry about table manners; these will take care of themselves if the child is not continually interfered with.

Both Spock and *Infant Care* agree in their advice to mothers to start weaning the infant to a cup at 5 months, simply because it may be hard to accomplish if put off until the latter part of the first year. As in other developmental matters, parents are advised to undertake this gradually and only in accordance with the child's readiness to accept it. Follow-up observations of the rooming-in Project babies indicate that many children do not give up the bottle readily, especially a bedtime or naptime bottle, until the end of the second or even third year.

The child in the United States begins to try to undress himself at the age of 1 to 1½ years. By 2 he is able to remove all his clothes, but it is not really until 3 years that he can dress himself, at least put on the easy things. This period of the child's learning calls for great patience and restraint on the part of parents.

As for toilet-training: bowel-control is said to come first in the

91

developmental order, but among the children under our observation there are quite a number of instances where bladder-control has been achieved before bowel-control.

Infant Care stresses the importance of waiting until the baby is ready to learn and explains to the mother how she may recognize the signs of readiness. 'Many babies are not ready to start learning bowel-control by the end of the first year. One and a half or two years is a much more common time for them to learn willingly.' In regard to bladder-control, *Infant Care* states 'Very few babies indeed are ready to start learning bladder control by the time they are a year old. In most cases it is better to make no effort at all in this direction until well along in the second year, or even later.' *Infant Care* cautions mothers that they can easily make trouble for themselves or the baby if they start training too early. 'A child can get to feeling that his mother is his enemy if she urges on him things he is not ready for. His whole relationship with her can be injured by forcing and pressure.'

Spock recognizes that many mothers of to-day have been influenced by their parents to believe in early toilet-training. He is accordingly somewhat more conservative in his advice for beginning bowel-training. Mothers, he says, should wait until their child is approaching at least one year. He, too, cautions against forcing the child, but admits that it may be first tried around 7 or 9 months when the child can sit up steadily alone. He presents an excellent exposition of the child's interest in his bowel function in the second year, and the need for mothers to handle this sympathetically, and discusses 'the bad effects of a fight over bowel-training.' He states that a child will usually train himself for bowel function between 18 and 24 months if no struggle has taken place. For training the child to bladder-control, Spock advises to 'Go at it easily, when he is ready.' He says children usually become dry by day between 1½ years and 2½ years, and by night anywhere from 1½ years to 4 years. It is noted by both our source books that girls learn a little earlier than boys to be toilet-trained.

These examples illustrate that advice in regard to bringing up infants in the U.S.A. is in a state of flux from rigid scheduling to general principles of flexibility. It is hoped that a happy medium may be found in which beneficial limitations on a child's activities can be carefully enough defined in relation to developmental factors, to give specific help to parents in the guidance of their children to a comfortable adaptation within the family and subsequently to the larger community outside the home.

CHILDBIRTH PATTERNS IN THE UNITED STATES

Edith B. Jackson

AS AN INTRODUCTION, it may be useful to repeat the facts about shifts in developmental and growth norms: 26 per cent of the children reported by Gesell and Thompson (11) in 1938 and 44 per cent of the children reported by Peatman and Higgons (21) in 1940 were walking at 52 weeks; Dr. Klatskin (15) reported in 1952 that 61 per cent of 184 New Haven babies coming from a wide range of parental and socio-economic backgrounds were walking at one year. I wish to emphasize that there was no attempt on the part of the doctors in this last series to urge early muscular performance, though one must assume the existence of the usual maternal competitive striving. On the contrary, it remains traditional for the medical profession to point out to parents the unwisdom of urging the child to walk before he is ready.

Dr. Klatskin noted that the children studied both by Gesell and Thompson, and by Peatman and Higgons were born before 1940 and apparently raised on fixed feeding regimes rather than by general self-regulation which existed in the Yale Project[1] group ('Rooming-in'). It is a possibility, as both Trainham and Gilliland (13) indicate, that the amount of parental handling, exercise and stimulation received by infants on self-regulated regimes is greater than that received by infants on strict schedules. Dr. Klatskin interpreted the findings in the Yale Project group in the light of changing paediatric methodology, with its advances in nutrition, in control of disease, and in understanding developmental needs.

The need for re-standardizing infant development scales is illustrated by Meredith's 1943 study of stature (19), which demonstrated that the average 2½-year-old child was taller in 1940 than in 1880. Hereditary and sociological factors are more directly comparable in the study of the Harvard sons of Harvard fathers, who are one inch taller than their fathers were at the same age. These studies point to the need for re-standardization of tests and procedures in a rapidly changing society.

Rooming-in has significance as a spearhead of a kind of revolution which is quietly taking place in medical, nursing, and parent education

[1] See footnote p. 88.

93

in the United States. Perhaps its chief importance lies in the turn of the tide of mechanistic methods in maternal care in favour of a more human approach. Between 1915 and 1940, in the United States, the place of childbirth shifted almost completely from home to hospital. Hospital methods, with all their rigidity, dominated infant care; and the practical exclusion of the father from his child during the neo-natal period interfered with the integration of the family unit. Separate care of mother and infant in the hospital made a dull routine of this work; it narrowed the horizon and dimmed the enthusiasm of doctors and nurses in training.

Realization of desires to bring mother and infant together in the hospital, had to be preceded in New Haven by extension of the hospital paediatric supervision of infants into the neo-natal period at home until time for Well Baby Conference[1] attendance, that is, for the six-week period after the mother took the child home from the hospital. In the New Haven Hospital a home visiting plan for paediatricians in training, on their two-month assignment to the nursery, was introduced in 1938 by Dr. Grover Powers, chief of the service, with the co-operation of the City Health Department and the present of an automobile from an interested colleague. Seeing the infant in his home surroundings immediately vitalized the paediatric interne's work. He saw for himself the importance of becoming acquainted with the mother before she left the hospital and gauging his advice in terms of the parental situation. It brought him into co-operative working relationship with community health agencies, especially the visiting nurse, and it gave to the visiting nurse a consistent plan of medical supervision instead of a rather haphazard one, allowing for the exchange of reports and periodic joint staff conferences for review of procedures. At that time the home delivery service of the hospital was practically defunct, and medical students no longer had any direct experience with the family situation at any time during their training.

In the same year, in New Haven, Mrs. Erikson wanted to have her baby with her in the hospital. The hospital's rules were against this, and the request was denied. However, she contracted an infectious illness shortly before the baby's birth, so was delivered in isolation, and the rules demanded that the infant be kept with the mother. It was also in this year that Dr. Margaret Mead, in New York, prevailed on Dr. Spock to circumvent the rigid feeding schedule of the hospital for her own child; and it was a year or two later that Mrs. Simsarian and her paediatrician, Dr. McClendon, in Washington, D.C., worked out a plan for taking care of her baby in the hospital on a self-demand schedule. This latter was in order to make

---

[1] Also termed 'Child Welfare' or 'Infant Welfare'.

reliable records of a baby's response to self-demand, and it was necessary to place the baby in the mother's room. The term 'rooming-in' had been coined by Dr. Gesell and first appeared in the literature and common use in 1943. Thus, around 1940, educated mothers, usually with some psychological orientation, began to make personal requests for a different type of maternal care, thus drawing the attention of the medical and nursing profession to the need for the revision of hospital maternity practice.

Support came from doctors working in child guidance clinics. Between 1915 and 1940, in the U.S.A., observations on the behaviour of children in connection with exacting and rigid regimes can be found scattered through case reports of behaviour problem children. Rigid attitudes developed as hospitals took over care of the newborn baby. Possible disadvantages were overlooked in the beneficial results of decreased morbidity and mortality. A generation elapsed, during which time child guidance clinics developed, before the clinical impression was formed that absolute strictness in the management of the infant and authoritarian medical advice to parents, based on rules and not on understanding of the dynamics of human behaviour, were in themselves contributing to the knotty problems of parent-child relationships.

It became important to get more systematic observations of infant behaviour in relation to influences playing upon it, and at the same time to train doctors, nurses, social workers and parents in the available knowledge of child development. This, in broad survey, is the background of the trend in the United States towards flexibility in maternal and infant care, and to the increasing use of newborn nurseries and Well Baby Conferences in medical education.

Between 1946 and 1950 there developed, in close succession, a number of separate centres where rooming-in was practised, in teaching, private and military hospitals. The idea took hold sufficiently so that in 1950 the *Encyclopaedia Britannica* asked for information about the number of hospitals which offered rooming-in facilities: the answer was—about forty. This seemed to be a promising advance for something which required re-orientation and reorganization of staff, and close integration of obstetric, paediatric, nursing, administrative, psychiatric, and social service interests.

Our experience has been that mothers have loved having their babies near them and their husbands to visit with the baby present, but to accomplish such an arrangement has meant a tremendous change and very careful planning in relation to hospital and State rules. Mothers have been extremely appreciative of the nurses' care and very particularly of the ready availability of nurse and doctor to answer questions. The fathers have been very appreciative of the opportunity to show their interest. The service offers a really gratifying experience to both nurses and doctors, because the mother and child are taken care of together, and mother and father are instructed together as much as is possible.

I want to stress the educational value of the rooming-in unit for the nurses and the doctors. We have two four-bed units with free access from cubicle to cubicle and a dining-table for each unit. With a policy of early ambulation, the mothers get up for meals on the second or third day. The paediatrician gives a so-called 'going home' talk, when the mothers are nearly ready to leave the hospital. He introduces the discussion by anticipating from experience the questions that are likely to come up with the mothers in their homes during the following few weeks. The discussion is then a give-and-take affair, and it is remarkable to see how much confidence the primiparous mothers gain by learning from the experience of other mothers, as well as from the professional adviser.

Prospective mothers very soon started asking questions about Grantly Dick Read's (22) book on childbirth, and with some of our earliest rooming-in mothers, we worked out a very satisfactory procedure so that when, about four months later, Dr. Dick Read visited the New Haven Hospital, Mrs. Helen Heardman, lent by the Maternity Centre of New York, had already instituted mothers' classes in relaxation and exercises.

After a short time the obstetric service, under the direction of Dr. Herbert Thoms, developed a programme of preparing mothers for childbirth, with which the aims of the Rooming-in Project were recognized to be closely interwoven. The essential aims in both programmes are to encourage the mother's active participation, to reduce anxiety, and to provide anticipatory guidance, respectively about changes to be expected during the course of pregnancy and labour, and changes to be expected in the child's reactions as he develops from one phase to another.

At first, the paediatricians in the pre-natal clinic were amazed at the relief which the mothers seemed to have in talking to them. Almost every interview ended with: 'Thank you, doctor, for the time you have given me.' Now the training programme includes, in addition to the nurses' classes, a series of four evening lectures for each group of patients, mothers and fathers together. There is opportunity for the mothers who want to nurse the babies to learn to express colostrum from the breast in the last few weeks of pregnancy as an aid to nursing. There have been lectures on nutrition, and there has already arisen the possibility of over-teaching the mothers.

Natural childbirth, as practised in the New Haven Hospital obstetric service, is based on the premise that childbirth is a normal process. The mother's conscious participation in the process is encouraged; she is kept informed about what is happening, she learns through relaxation and through breathing to minimize the amount of discomfort. If a mother feels the need of relief from pain, or if the obstetrician feels she should have relief, he provides for the appropriate treatment, sedation, anaesthesia or assistance in completing the birth. The mother, however, is not drugged, she actively participates during most of the delivery, and is usually able to see her child immediately after birth.

There is general agreement among obstetricians throughout the United States that episiotomy is a beneficial procedure, and it is routinely performed in many hospitals. Natural spontaneous deliveries do not necessarily occur without tears, and when tears do occur, they may be ragged, deep, and difficult to repair. They do not heal as quickly as a short incision which can be neatly and quickly repaired with no extra discomfort for the mother at the time of the infant's delivery. The doctor tells mothers who are conscious that he is going to inject a little novocaine and make a slight cut, so that the delivery of the head will be easier and possible without anaesthetic. At that point in delivery, the stretching of the tissues is so great that there is very little sensation. The incision is then neatly repaired immediately after delivery, while the effects of the novocaine are still present.

The use of elective forceps is quite frequent in general obstetric practice. Many obstetricians consider that when the head is presenting and making extremely slow progress, it is better for both baby and mother to ease delivery by the application of low forceps. This procedure has been used less frequently at the New Haven Hospital since the institution of the 'Training for Childbirth' programme.

It should be emphasized that the Yale Project cases were selected in order to illustrate a method of study of parent-child relationship, with particular reference to the degree of flexibility of parental attitude in child care. The fact that all three of the cases presented to the Seminar in one way or another presented a somewhat unstable picture is coincidental. The U.S.A. has its share of healthy, mature and stable mothers who can love and discipline their children without undue anxiety and guilt.

The question was raised as to why more was not done to help one of our mothers.[1] During her college education, this mother had become imbued with the importance of rooming-in facilities and flexible regimes. She felt so strongly about certain things that she could not always follow her paediatrician's advice. Because of her interest in the study, she volunteered to make occasional reports to

[1] Avis: a case studied at the Seminar, but not included in Vol. II.

the rooming-in paediatricians, although it was clearly understood they were not supervising her care of the child. When the child was 9 months old, her mother voluntarily sought a psychiatrist's advice on a specific question in relation to leaving the child, and accepted his recommendations. If she had returned with further questions, indicating an awareness of a problem with which she needed help, the possibility of therapy would certainly have been discussed, but without any further indication on the mother's part of need for help, he did not feel in a position to impose suggestions for therapy. ·

Another mother got as far as asking for and receiving definite advice to get psychiatric treatment for herself, but she turned it down. There are many factors involved in the possibility of helping mothers of which one of the most important factors is, of course, a readiness to be helped. In the meantime, the nursery school teachers, guided by psychiatric consultation, will try to offer the child a favourable emotional 'climate' for the development of his best potentialities.

The Yale study is a kind of hybrid because, at the outset, we were equally interested in the clinical and educational aspects of the rooming-in programme. Careful consideration was given to the welfare and comfort of each mother and infant in the rooming-in unit through the integration of the obstetric, paediatric and nursing staffs. The research project derived its name from the rooming-in unit which, *per se*, offered a unique opportunity for staff members to observe mother and child together. But it was the general framework of the research plan which offered education and training, particularly for paediatricians. Two or three paediatricians were appointed annually to work full time with the Rooming-in Project. It was a new development to have paediatricians in training devote so much time to work with well babies only. The paediatricians conducted pre-natal interviews to get experience of the mother's attitude, as she looked forward to the baby's arrival and her responsibility in caring for it. They came to realize the eagerness of mothers for help at this time, and the importance of their getting it.

It was soon found that during these interviews complicated problems would sometimes come up which the paediatricians did not know how to handle. The questionnaire method was devised to help with the interview and as a guide to bring out points which experience had already shown most mothers wanted to discuss. Moreover, the standard questionnaires were important for providing comparable data.

The rapport which the paediatrician gained with the mothers in the pre-natal clinic helped him when the mothers came to the hospital. He could thus follow the development of the mother-child relationship in the hospital, in the home during the first two months, at the six-week check-up, and, in a number of cases, in the Well Baby Conference, to which the mothers bring the children once a month during the first year. Here they are seen first by the visiting nurse (or health visitor) and then the physician, for the discussion of any points which the nurse or the mother wish to have clarified. The experience of advising numerous mothers about their infants, month after month, leads the paediatrician-in-training to face a problem, which will later confront him in practice, viz., that his capacity to give appropriate help may sometimes be limited by the unwillingness or unconscious inability of some mothers to follow advice.

DISCUSSION

Some of the American studies of child development were started more than twenty years ago. In 1926-7 Lawrence K. Frank, then with the Rockefeller-Spellman Foundation, planned long-term research in child development, and also set aside funds for the training of personnel and to educate the lay public in backing up the teachers. The spontaneous movement which has led to rooming-in, self-regulation, and so on, was an outcome of that planning, and now that in many countries people are embarking on this type of research, it is valuable to emphasize the usefulness of a multiple programme, to include training and education.

It is perhaps true that the particular kind of institutionalism which entailed the birth of babies in hospitals, anaesthetics, forceps, disposing of the mother for the convenience of the doctors, keeping her in bed, and artificial feeding, went further in America than anywhere else. There is now a reaction in America against those very practices which are spreading over the rest of the world, through personnel trained in America. One must recognize the importance of these battles in certain countries, in the hope that they will not have to be fought elsewhere.

There are other possible effects of rapid change in child care advice. To teach mothers to treat their third or fourth child in a completely different way from their first child may create serious maternal anxiety, she may wonder what harm she has done to the older child. It is extremely important to spread over the country the kind of infant care which could make it unnecessary to attempt to reverse the situation later.

However, one must avoid the mistake of oversimplifying 'good' and 'bad' in training, for to do so may make the mothers feel guilty and helpless. It may be more important that obstetricians and paediatricians are being converted to 'natural childbirth' in conjunction with modern scientific methods.

99

The main contribution of rooming-in has been, as emphasized, that of an educational device, and its modification of medical and nursing education and procedure, for example, the 'case assignment' of the nurse, rather than the 'job assignment'.

Self-regulation, itself, may vary. For instance, a mother may feed her child at certain scheduled times, but she may give him something to eat when he is hungry, pick him up when he cries, and have fun in playing with him. This is not following a strict schedule at all, and such observations illustrate how relatively unimportant all these theories are and how important it is to help the mother to feel comfortable and natural. A mother who becomes over-anxious may damage her child. A mother must be able to express her love and affection for her child comfortably.

In the U.S.A., arrangements for the care of children under 5 when the mother goes to hospital vary, according to the individual family circumstances. Very often a grandmother, or other relative or a neighbour comes to help. Sometimes the children are sent to their grandparents or relatives. Children under 16 are not allowed to visit in the hospital, and the question arises of the separation of the toddler from his mother. The shortening of the hospital period and the increased readiness of father to take over the supervision of the toddler reduce the possible trauma. Many fathers plan their vacations for the time of the expected delivery, so as to look after the child at home.

Some public and voluntary social agencies are developing a homemaker's service of trained people to go into a home and cook and care for the other children while the mother is in the hospital.

Other countries are not strictly comparable with the U.S.A.; for example, in the U.K. rooming-in has perhaps never been entirely lost, and indeed, hospital confinements constitute no more than one-half of the whole. The centre of the struggle in Britain is neither the well baby nor 'natural' childbirth in hospital: it concerns the relationship between the whole family and the sick child. In Denmark, 95 to 96 per cent of the population are members of a sickness club and can have their family doctor free. Pregnant women have five examinations by their own doctor and six or seven examinations by a midwife. In Yugoslavia, the fight for hygiene, sanitation, and mental health is at its beginning. It has been found best not to make too many rules, but to leave the mother free to develop her own initiative. Mothers are told that they should never give a baby anything that they have not tried themselves and that the quality must be good, but that quantity must be determined by circumstances.

Part Three

STUDIES OF INFANT

RELATIONSHIP FORMATION

CHILDHOOD DEVELOPMENT PHENOMENA

THE INFLUENCE OF THE MOTHER-CHILD RELATIONSHIP, AND ITS DISTURBANCES

René Spitz

THERE IS an impression that in investigations into babyhood, the problem of emotions is excluded because of the exactness of the observations. That need not be so; this whole investigation is centred around the emotional life of the child. The two most important turning-points in the emotional life of the child during the first year of life are the third month and the eighth month. In the third month the emotional maturation of the infant is the pioneer, the trail-breaker, for every other development in that infant's life. The infant recognizes a person—his mother or her substitute—because of his emotional tie to her, but not the rest of the world because such ties have not yet been developed; the emotions linking him with the rest of the world are not strong enough. It is an axiom that emotional understanding precedes other understanding by at least two months, throughout the first year of life. The infant recognizes his mother at 3 months and the bottle or its food only at 5 or 6 months. The infant distinguishes the mother from a stranger usually between the sixth and eighth months, but it distinguishes its favourite toy only towards 10 months. Its disappointment when somebody who has been playing with it goes away, is already visible at 4 months; but if you take away a toy, disappointment will only become visible after 6 months.

The film Grief[1] was made because of my conviction of the central importance of the mother-child relationship.

Why is the mother so important for the child? Of course, she gives the child not only comfort, but support—everything—and the mother's importance is in direct proportion to the helplessness of the infant throughout the first year. The more helpless the infant the more important the role of the mother, or of the person who fulfils the role of the mother.

[1] Grief, A Peril in Infancy. See Film List, p. 297.

Now it is difficult to understand the mother-child relationship unless you are a mother yourself or have watched it pretty closely. It is quite a specific attachment—a form of behaviour which is centred solely on one being. Perhaps the best illustration of what this means can be seen in the case of the mother suckling her baby, for whom the rest of the world has simply vanished. Suckling is the focus of her whole personality and in this, the role of the immediate skin to skin contact is infinitely important, though nearly completely lost in Western cultures. We have isolated ourselves from our children by layers of cloth, sterility, asepsis and caution. I have a suspicion that many of the psychogenic diseases in Western cultures have something to do with this loss of skin to skin contact between mother and suckling child.

From the premise that the mother-child relation is supremely important, I investigated what forms it took, in an environment which was particularly suited to the purposes of study—a penal nursery environment. There were about fifty children whom I could see regularly over a year or more, with their mothers; and whenever I saw some change in a child I had an opportunity to relate it to what happened to the mother.

One day we found a child, who had previously smiled back at us in the most charming fashion, not doing so, but getting scared. This started a further investigation, during which the total of subjects observed over a long term was 366, and of those 256 were observed over six months. They came from six different environments: a nursery, private homes, foster homes, a foundling home, a maternity hospital and a native village.

In the nursery in which I made the film, a succession of doctors saw the children weep and slowly fade and did not realize why: but the matron recognized the reason clearly, because she was naturally endowed with that kind of maternal feeling which enabled her to sense what went on. When I asked her 'What is the matter with Jane?', she said, 'Well, her mother has left her.' Before training nurses, an effort should be made to enable them to get into touch with children and to understand them naturally in the way in which they would if they were their own children.

Why is the mother so important? Theoretically it is possible to say that in the beginning, all learning on the part of the child is in the form of the conditioned reflex. It is only later, after a psychic organization has been developed, that learning takes place in another manner. With a conditioned reflex bewilderment occurs if the least little item of the stimulus is changed. What the child experiences with the mother has the effect of a conditioner. What acts on the child at this earliest stage are the mother's emotions, her feelings, the

104

interchange of these with the child's responses and the effect of the child's responses on the mother's feelings. The inter-relation between mother and child in the first two months is essentially an emotional one.

When the mother is taken away from this child, it loses the very foundations of its existence. It now has to adjust to completely alien circumstances in a manner which no grown-up can imagine, because nothing—or hardly anything—can happen which will put an adult in the hopeless situation of a child whose whole world, comprised of its mother, disappears. Her replacement is then of paramount importance. If the replacing person has a special, intimate understanding of the child, then, after very brief contacts, she will feel what the child wants; she will give contact when the child wants contact and she will not force contact when the child does not want it. There was one person in whose arms children did not weep, and that was the matron of whom I spoke. That matron could go in to any child in the deepest depression, weeping, screaming, or anything, take it in her arms, and in a few moments that child was reassured.

The symptoms of maternal deprivation after the age of 6 months are progressive. In the first month of separation, the child shows the weeping, demanding attitude shown at the beginning of the film *Grief*;[1] it is as if the child were reaching out for another person. In the second month the child shows withdrawal, and if you do approach it, it begins to scream; it begins to lose weight and the developmental quotient falls. In the third month of separation the child takes up the characteristic position of lying flat on its belly; it withdraws and does not want contact with the world; if it is disturbed it screams incessantly. I observed one such child screaming for three hours, stopping only to catch its breath. It begins to suffer from severe insomnia, loses weight, becomes a prey to intercurrent ailments and infections, becomes accident-prone and has cuts, scratches, bruises and other skin troubles.

In the fourth month of separation the facial expression becomes rigid, screaming ceases and the child begins to wail. Now the developmental quotient falls quickly. The social sector, however, remains high. With three months' separation the developmental quotient regresses, on the average, 12½ points; from three to four months it regresses 14 points, and over five months it regresses 25 points.

The separated child also loses previously acquired skills; for example, if it had already been able to stand in its crib and to walk around by holding on, after the mother goes away it will stop walking and standing and not even sit up any more. It loses faculties

[1] See Film List, p. 297.

which it had already acquired, for in due time a refusal to perform amounts to a loss of those faculties, because they cannot be regained.

Children who have been separated for less than three months will regain their faculties within a few days of the mother's return; but separation for a longer period has more lasting effects.

In the case of children to whom the mothers return after about three months, the developmental quotient takes a jump within the week of the mother's return, and the child suddenly becomes gay, happy and active.

Separations of mother and child lasting longer than three months, without adequate substitution, are no longer to be found in institutions in the United States. Therefore, I had to go to another country where I found an institution, a foundling home, housing ninety-one infants separated from their mothers for periods of longer duration.

Under three months of separation the quotient gains after reunion, on the average, 25 points; if the separation is somewhat longer, some 13 points; if it has been still longer, rather less; and with over five months of separation it not only does not gain but the regression continues. Regression has now become a progressive process and special measures will be needed (if special measures can help at all) to get these children back. Up to three months, reversible changes occur; from three to five months is the critical transition period, and after a period of over five months of separation the changes tend to become irreversible.

The influence of deprivation on the weight of the children is considerable. Normally, a child reaches fifteen to seventeen pounds around 10 months, whereas deprived children take 2 years and 6 months to reach this weight. These children take $3\frac{1}{2}$ years to reach the weight of twenty-five pounds, as compared with the normal time of 1 year and 1 month.

More important as criteria, however, are the child's activities and skills. I observed the children in the institution for a total of two years, by which time most of them had reached the age of 4 years. At 4 years, of the original ninety-one, twenty-one remained, of whom five could not walk at all; sixteen walked by holding on to the furniture; twelve could not eat alone with a spoon; twenty could not dress alone—only one could; six were not toilet-trained at all, and the other fifteen showed only a minimal response to toilet-training. Six of the children could not talk at all, five had a vocabulary of two words, one a dozen words, and one actually spoke in sentences.

The one child who could speak, walk, dress itself, and eat alone, and who was toilet-trained, was of an angelic beauty—just like an angel by Raphael—and no person who came into that nursery failed to stop at the child's bed and talk and play with it. Every nurse stooped down to tickle its chin, every doctor stopped and spoke to it, and so this was the one child among these foundling home children who really did get something in the nature of emotional interchange with another human being. All the other children, after the third month, were reared by a nurse who did not have the time to do anything more than feed the ten or twelve who were in her charge. Accordingly she stuck the bottle in the child's mouth and rushed away to the next child. There was no opportunity for any contact with the children, and as this process progressed, the facial expression of each child became rigid, frozen, immobile, far-away and dazed, and the weeping subsided completely.

The paediatrician in charge said to me at my first visit: 'The children do not cry here. It is very strange, the children are so extra-ordinarily quiet. Even if you perform an operation like perforating the ear-drum, they only cry a little and then stop suddenly.' In that ward in which approximately fifty children were lying, there was a deathly silence; on rare occasions did you hear one child weeping. This situation is quite characteristic. In our hospitals, parents are distressed by the child's weeping when the parents leave, and the nurse says: 'Oh well, you cannot visit your child for the next few weeks, but if you come back after four weeks the child will be quiet and will have become accustomed to it.' Yes, it will be quiet, but it may be the silence of death.

Of the ninety-one children whom we observed in the foundling home, thirty-two were placed in families or other institutions, and we lost track of them completely. Of four we have no records. I have just given a report of how the twenty-one who stayed in the home looked at four years of age. They might just as well have died. Then there is the terrible figure of $37\frac{1}{2}$ per cent who did die in the course of two years.

These results can be contrasted with those of the penal nursery, in which the children were raised with their own mothers. In the course of five years' observation there was not a single major infec-tious epidemic and no deaths, though, in the penal nursery, the children were less of a random selection than the foundling home children, for they were the children of delinquent, criminal, feeble-minded mothers and of mothers with a bad heredity.

The penal nursery was well-run and clean as things go, but not compulsively so about cleanliness and hand-washing and so on. If I washed my hands on arrival it was fine, but nobody paid much attention; if I put on a white coat it was wonderful, but street clothes were all right too. Nurses came in from outside, and still no epidemic developed and no deaths ensued.

On the other hand, the foundling home was a very hygienic place.

The moment I stepped in at the door I was shown into a cubicle with two disinfectants to wash my hands, and then a nurse threw a white coat over me. The children were visited daily by the head physician, and every afternoon by various specialists as necessary, but epidemic after epidemic swept through that place. This is a vivid illustration of the vital importance of the presence of a mother-figure with the children.

DISCUSSION

Undoubtedly the conditions in the particular nursery under observation could have been improved by conducting the nursery differently, such as by having more nurses and one nurse devoting herself to two or three infants. That particular nursery was selected because it seemed that there could be no worse emotional conditions in which to raise infants. Physically they were not deprived but emotionally they were very seriously so.

At the start of the observation no child in the nursery had a toy. They lay in their beds day in and day out, they could not move themselves and they were not moved. The observers all had strict instructions to observe and not to advise; to evade questions, as otherwise they would influence the experiment.

The result, however, of their mere presence in the institution over a number of months evoked some reaction in the staff, and slowly, here and there a toy began to appear on a child's bed, until by the end of the period nearly every child had a toy suspended somewhere. After three months a disused cage which had been there all the time was placed on a verandah in the sun, and about a dozen children carried out there.

Under such horrible circumstances giving the child even a slight chance of other stimulation would enable it to form something of a personality. If a person lay in a bed and had to look at a ceiling and nothing else, what could one expect that person to become?

The two nurseries presented an extremely contrasting picture, and it must be left to the imagination of observers to visualize how the whole gamut of deprivation may start.

CHILDHOOD DEVELOPMENT PHENOMENA

THE CASE OF FELICIA[1]

René Spitz

FELICIA was brought up in the nursery of a prison, where children were looked after by their prisoner mothers, supervised by professional trained nurses. The institution, as institutions for babies go, was excellent. There were no fathers. The mothers were there for various reasons, mainly because of sexual delinquency, under the so-called Wayward Minors Act, but there were many other delinquents, such as thieves, and even murderers. Felicia's mother was a sexual delinquent, but not a prostitute.

A series of weekly observations of Felicia and her mother during the whole of the first year of Felicia's life, revealed that the child in a curious manner changed her behaviour, remarkably parallel with certain changes in her mother.

Various sectors of the capacity of the child were studied, viz., perception, body mastery capacity, mastery of social relations, learning (which brought in both imitation and memory), manipulation of objects, and finally, intelligence. At the age of 1 month and 2 days, at which the investigation started, one can measure the capacity for perception, for body mastery, and for social relations and learning. Later, by the eighth or tenth month, body mastery can be measured by offering the child, who is sitting, two objects at the same time. It will also crawl along. On the social relations side, the child who is approached in an active manner will show anxiety; it will shake hands, understanding that this is a social gesture; and if you turn your back it will try to get back into contact with you.

As to memory, if you cover an object with a piece of paper, it will uncover it. It can imitate your gestures. As for handling of materials, if it is given two spoons, it will hit them one against the other. On the intellectual side, if you place its favourite toy before it with some other object, the baby will grasp the toy; and if you change the position of the two objects it will do so again.

From these observations we get a figure for each of the sectors

[1] A case studied at the Seminar, but not included in Vol. II.

and also a total figure for the development quotient. The development quotient which we ascertain by this means does not represent absolute measure, but is rather a mode of comparison.

Felicia at the age of 1 month and 27 days was somewhat deficient. At 4 months and 13 days the child showed a striking disparity between the different sectors, which is unusual. Her social behaviour, though seemingly deficient, showed striking discrepancies with the social behaviour of children of that age in general; she did not, for example, respond to the grown-up's smile by smiling back. I have made a film of the smiling responses of a baby.[1] In this film we confront children with investigators whom they see for the first time; the child is slightly bewildered by the stranger but smiles immediately. The colour of the stranger makes no difference. The negro baby smiles at white people and the white baby smiles at coloured people. Racial discrimination is not inborn.

In a further sequence of the film, it is seen that the observer grimaces but the emotional stimulus (the friendly smile) is not offered to the child. The adult might think the face funny but I do not think the baby does. Then we have ascertained the response of the baby to masked faces—faces wearing Hallowe'en masks and with the tongue protruding through the mask's mouth. The infant responded to this and other grimaces with the same welcoming smile as it shows to any adult. As for inanimate objects, the child on being presented with a bottle, shows that it wants to drink but it does not smile.

At 4 months, Felicia did not respond to a smiling face by a smile but, paradoxically, by a scream. Screaming is also a recognition of the human factor; the human face presented to a baby may be a signal for relief or for unhappiness. Breast-fed babies as soon as they can open their eyes look at the mother's face during the feeding. This baby responded to the human face at times by screaming, and this, although negative, is still a social reaction, that is, one of reciprocity.

We therefore inquired more closely into the child's relations with her mother, and learnt that Felicia's mother had attached herself to another girl (Bertha) in the prison. Bertha was a severe psychopath with criminal tendencies and the attachment between the two girls was of a homosexual nature for which Bertha had a capacity. She would incite the girls attached to her to riot against the institution.

Felicia's mother became her submissive slave. Bertha influenced these girls to neglect or ill-treat their children. The matron of the institution then attempted a heart-to-heart talk with Felicia's mother and succeeded in winning her over. Two weeks later, I found Felicia

[1] *The Smiling Response.* See Film List, p. 297.

in the hands of her mother and the baby's reaction to my face was outgoing and friendly, like that of normal children. For disciplinary reasons, Bertha had been taken out of the nursery and so the evil influence was removed, but this was not to endure. Bertha returned, and Felicia's mother again fell under Bertha's spell.

At 5 months and 18 days the paradoxical social reaction again appeared in Felicia, and, in addition, there was retardation in the factor of learning. The matron, who saw this development, again tried talking with the mother and luckily once more Bertha had to be removed for disciplinary reasons and Felicia's mother became attached to the matron and proud of her own child. The baby returned to the normal smiling response, and there was an increase in the development quotient. Learning, however, was relatively retarded and perception absolutely so, as before. These responses of Felicia were very different from those of a normal child; it was not easy to establish contact; and it was not easy to get her to respond to an observer, particularly a female.

As an experiment, I approached Felicia with two female observers. Felicia responded by crying. I lifted Felicia up in my arms and she turned to the two female observers and cried more strongly, then looked at me and cried a little less. I put her down and crying ceased. I then went back alone to Felicia and from time to time she smiled. At this point two female prisoners came in and she immediately started to scream. She was again left alone and then I came back alone, smiled at her, and she answered with a smile. This was repeated three times and each time it worked. Then I called in the two female observers and left Felicia with them. She immediately started to scream. Finally, I sent in one female observer alone and Felicia answered by crying. The presence of several persons, particularly female, seemed to be a threat to Felicia, and in view of her mother's relations with Bertha, I think the child's behaviour can easily be interpreted: that the child had had imprinted on her, as a signal of danger, a female person.

The next four weeks passed peacefully. The mother had no relations with the other girls and the effect of the mother's improvement was strikingly visible in the child. Her development quotient went up to 131. In her social relations she achieved a level equal to that of a 1-year-old child when she was only 7 months and 20 days. She seemed able to participate in social interchange, and her inhibitions or whatever the painful experience may have been, seemed to have been overcome. It is questionable indeed whether these past bad experiences had not acted in some way as a stimulant of development of much further discrimination than is usually shown at that age.

Once again, unfortunately, Bertha regained her ascendancy over the mother and immediately the relation between mother and child deteriorated. At 8 months and 25 days Felicia's development quotient, which at 7 months and 20 days was 131, had fallen to 101. She had lost the whole of the advance she had made in the previous two months. She lagged behind in the social sector and in the manipulation of objects, and so far as the remaining sectors were concerned, she had lost the previous advance.

At this point both Bertha and the mother were removed because a really serious riot had broken out. Two weeks after the departure of the mother, when she was 9 months and 9 days old, Felicia was making moaning sounds; she was not interested in a doll which was brought her and she would not take up contacts any more. A week later she began to cry whenever she was approached, but when we left the room she looked after us with interest, though she cried when we came back.

She remained separated from her mother for two and a half months, during which time she produced all the behaviour patterns which are characteristic of a mother-child separation. She reached out for human fellowship: she missed her mother, but what she missed was not an all-encompassing relationship such as a normal child has.

When she was 11 months and 15 days old her mother returned. Two days later, when she was filmed, she appeared to be an energetic, happy child.

Large-scale studies have shown that children who had been in good relations with their mothers produced, on separation, a really severe reaction in 65.5 per cent, a mild reaction in 27 per cent, and no reaction in 7.5 per cent; whereas children who prior to the separation had been in bad relations with their mothers showed no reaction after separation in 71 per cent, a mild reaction in 29 per cent, and none of them a severe reaction.

The consequences of the relationship between mother and child and of the changes and disturbances in that relationship are well illustrated in the case of Felicia. Her mother was capable of making good relations with her child and Felicia's development was good so long as the relations remained at that level. But the mother was a labile character who could be influenced intimately by another.

The closeness of the relations between mother and child is mirrored in the child's personality step by step: I might almost speak of it as a mother-child binomial. Just as the mother influences the way in which the child behaves and develops, so in the same way, the child in its turn influences the mother and provokes in her action and reaction which, in turn again, will influence the child. But in this there is the difference that the mother is a grown-up with a well-established personality, and therefore has means at her hands of dealing with her reactions, which the child does not possess. Thus the mother's reaction will be relatively a partial one, a milder one.

The reaction of the child might go to fatal lengths, as was the experience with a group of children who had been breast-fed by their own mothers during the first three months of life and then separated and entrusted to the care of nursing personnel. The result was catastrophic, for in the course of two years the proportion of children who died was 37.5 per cent. The first investigation along these lines was made in 1910 by the Prussian Ministry of Health, Prussia at that time being probably the most hygienic country in the world. There it was discovered that the mortality in the course of the first year in institutions which had children without mothers, reached, in one case, a maximum of 71 per cent.

DISCUSSION

In order to ascertain whether the women in the penal institution were good or bad mothers, a very simple method was used. Every Saturday the mothers had a film show for three hours, during which time they were away from their children. At the end of that time the mothers re-appeared in droves and the observers stood and watched their reactions; a good mother would go to her child and cuddle it and see whether it was comfortable and dry; an indifferent mother might go to the smoking-room for a quiet smoke and not even bother to see whether her child still existed; and a bad mother would rush straight into her child's cubicle and would yell 'Who touched my child? Who did this or that to my child?' while ministering to her child so roughly that it would end up by screaming.

Dr. Spitz said: 'I once compared an unselected sample of children in an institution with a sample of private family children in families where the mother-child relation was good.

One interesting outcome was the similarity between the developmental curve of a family child who developed a behavioural disturbance and that of the institution child. The mother had certain qualities which exerted a damaging influence on the child. The developmental curve was characteristic of children on whom one specific factor is acting.

The smiling experiment was conducted over a couple of years on about 150 children. At birth the visual perception of the child is practically non-existent; the first ascertainable visual perception occurs somewhere in the second month, but there is as yet no reciprocal response of the child. Around 6 weeks the child, who does not pay any attention to any toy offered him, will stare at the human face and follow its movements. At that age, and up to about

6 months, the child does not perceive food. Emotional development precedes perceptual development. The latter proceeds in distinct phases, for example in the perception of food: at first the food is recognized only when the nipple is introduced into the mouth; by the fifth day the child recognizes the feeding situation—i.e., if the child is put in the feeding position it immediately turns its head towards the person who has put it into that position, and tries to suck. The next step is that the hungry child changes its behaviour at the moment when somebody approaches—its first distance perception, but appearing only as a function of the child's inner need, not as a function of the actual perception. In the next step, apart from feeding, the child recognizes any object approached to its face and promptly begins to move its mouth and tries to suck. At the third month the child recognizes a pointed object, but it is 6 months before it will recognize a bottle with a white liquid, as food.

Examination of the smiling response shows that what the child recognizes is a privileged *Gestalt*, consisting of a nose, two eyes and a forehead, in movement. In one of the first experiments which I made in Vienna, at a receiving station for infants, staffed by women, the children smiled at the women but not at me. Although tempted to theorize about the differences of sex, I looked at my reflection in the mirror and realized that the difference might be that the women had hair and I had not! When I had taken off my glasses and put on a little black cap, all the children smiled at me.

In an attempt to simplify the constituent elements of the *Gestalt* involved, we tried to find out whether it was really the eyes that mattered. On covering the mouth the child still smiled but not when the eyes were covered. On covering one eye, the smiling again stopped. The conclusion was that two eyes, a nose, a forehead and movement were needed. Without movement, the child would not only not smile but would get a progressively more frightened expression on its face.

In these experiments there was no other kind of stimulus than the visual, and the child was not touched. No differentiation had been made between smiling and laughing because it had not seemed sufficiently important for the purposes of this particular perceptual reaction. It would be very important to make such a differentiation for the purpose of investigating emotional development, but this comes later. Delays in smiling were due to individual differences of the children, and had nothing to do with either the mask or face. The children reacted with the same readiness to either, but some of the more advanced children became bewildered when they were shown either face or mask, whereas others who were not as advanced smiled more readily.

114

The face is the first visual percept, but in order of appearance of percepts a child reacts to position first, then to touch, then to hearing and then, about four weeks later, to a visual percept. The sense of smell does not seem to play a role in the child's life at that early age. Children presented with the breast of a woman with milk expressed on the nipple and brought under their noses do not change their behaviour. The claim that smell is one of the earliest percepts seems to have been proved only for extreme smells, such as ammonia, and not the smell of food.'

.　　　.　　　.　　　.　　　.

Dr. Spitz then showed a film[1] dealing with relations between mother and child, and the reactions of various children to their mothers' attitudes at feeding.

The mother's behaviour favours the retention of the necessary patterns of behaviour and the discarding of the unnecessary and useless ones. Thus in an almost intangible manner the mother gives the child the direction in which it is to develop in the course of the first year.

There are a few experimental investigations which have appeared to show that in the first year of life, month by month, breast-fed infants within the same environment are more advanced in their mental development than bottle-fed infants. Bodily development may be relatively more advanced in bottle-fed infants than in the breast-fed infant, the theory being that mental development can only occur as a result of emotional stimulation by the environment, which in this case is the mother; the woman reacts to what the infant does to her breast and the circular relationship is fulfilled exactly.

Dr. Spitz said that the smiling response is quite specific and not just smiling in general; reference to children of 26 days giving the smiling response meant specifically the *response*. Any parent knows perfectly well that children smile much earlier than that. The earliest is possibly at 3 or 6 days, or even from the first day, but such a smile is a motor overflow and not a specific response expression: it might equally well smile as kick its legs, or scream. The best method used by experimental psychologists to ascertain this point, is to see whether there is any significant difference between the number of times the child smiles without any kind of stimulation and when it is shown something. Up to the time of the acquisition of the real response smile, statistics show that the smile is just a recurring movement of muscles which are available to the child——a fact which was perfectly well known by our grandmothers, who used to say that when a child smiled it had the wind.

[1] *Mother–Child Relations.* See Film List, p. 297.

It is a common practice in hospital for mothers to wear masks when they feed their babies, and experiments are needed to support, or otherwise, the feeling that this is not a sound practice. Merely to cover the lower part of the face does not matter, but a mask reaching up to the eyes might have a harmful effect. With regard to the nurses in hospitals all wearing masks, there comes a time around the age of 6 months when the child begins to distinguish friend from stranger, and all the stimulus which a child can get from the face becomes more important because, in recognizing faces, more than just the eyes, nose and forehead is used, and hence the mask is probably not a good thing.

It is sometimes questioned whether, when myelinization of the brain is not complete, one is justified in speaking of intellect; but it is a fact that children acquire intellectual insight long before myelinization has taken place, and this acquisition can be retarded or stopped by inappropriate behaviour on the part of the mother.

The film[1] of mothers feeding their babies showed one mother who was giving herself to her baby in a sort of rapture, but who was wearing a nipple-shield; and this appears to show that even such a handicap as an inverted or insufficient nipple does not preclude the mother's giving herself completely to the baby and feeding it, although one might have thought it to be a very considerable bar to the formation of good relationships. Perhaps it might be concluded that love passes all understanding and overcomes all obstacles.

[1] *Mother–Child Relations.* See Film List, p. 297.

MOTHER–CHILD SEPARATION

John Bowlby

WHAT IS MEANT by mental ill-health? To me, at least, the most concrete concept of mental ill-health is a derangement of the capacity to make co-operative relationships with other human beings. Medical studies and pathology are concerned with function and dysfunction, of which psychiatrists study in particular the capacity to make relationships with other people. This is not the whole of psychiatry, but it is, in a sense, its centre, and a very large proportion of psychiatric troubles are manifestly defects in the capacity to make relationships.

What constitutes the normal human capacity to make relationships? To define the norm in regard to social relationships raises the question of anthropological relativities, since what is the social norm in one culture is not so in another. Nevertheless, there are certain common patterns: a certain minimal nexus of social relationships must exist if a culture is to survive. For instance, if an adult cannot make a certain relationship with a member of the opposite sex the process of reproduction is not able to begin, and if he or she cannot make a certain relationship with a baby, reproduction cannot continue. It is perhaps only about 6,000 years ago that man attempted the task of going beyond these basic, biological, family relationships to form larger societies. It is evident that he still has much to learn about how to achieve this, but the realization that these extended relationships are developments from the simpler family relationships is vital for success in the larger enterprise.

We can therefore distinguish two main sorts of relationship—family (or love) relationships and extended relationships. In the sphere of love relationships, the mentally ill person is at his worst. The neurotic person may or may not be difficult as employer or employee, but his love relationships are always unsatisfactory, and this applies equally to the psychotics. Indeed, following a breakdown in a love relationship people often develop a psychosis. Again, the psychopathic personality is unable to make any continuous co-operative love relationship, but moves from one potential love object to another.

Thus the study of love relationships and their dysfunction is at the centre of the psychiatrist's study. It is a basic proposition of psychoanalysis that these family relationships—the child-parent relationship, the husband-wife relationship, and the parent-child relationship—have much in common; that the kind of child-parent relationship which a person experienced in his childhood is reflected in his later relationship to husband or wife and to children. In child guidance it is found not only that maladjusted children have parents who are making many mistakes with them, but that these mistakes derive from unconscious attitudes which stem from the parents' own childhood.

Because this central proposition has often been challenged, it is particularly interesting that similar conclusions have been reached by students of animal behaviour—I refer especially to the group of ethologists headed by Konrad Lorenz and Niko Tinbergen. They have established that organisms are born with certain innate instinctive social responses which are normally directed towards members of their own species, but that precise development of these responses may depend in very high degree on the individual's experience at certain critical phases of his life. Thus in the normal course of events, the gosling's 'following-response' becomes directed towards mother goose so that the young goose remains as closely attached to its mother as any 2-year-old human infant. Later on, too, its mating response is directed towards a bird of its own species of the opposite sex. However, the goose *may* become fixated on a human being instead of its mother, whilst there is the sad case of the peacock which wooed only tortoises. How do these fixations develop? The gosling's following-response is elicited by the first fairly large moving object seen by the newly hatched bird. Normally, of course, this is the mother, but fixations can occur to a variety of objects, some singularly unfitted to mother the young bird (Lorenz) (16). In the case of the sexual response there is a further complication, in that the object to which the sexual response is directed may be imprinted long before the sexual response has become fully active. Thus the object to which a peacock will display may be determined by the objects which he meets in the first weeks or months after hatching. If, as in one case, the peacock is brought up in the reptile house of a zoo, his sexual responses may be irrevocably turned towards an object as unsuitable as a giant tortoise (Lorenz) (17).

That later love relationships in birds can be profoundly influenced by earlier experiences is now abundantly proven. Less work has been done with mammals but enough is known to make it clear that the position is not wholly different. Thus if a lamb is brought up in a farmhouse, all its social responses become directed towards human beings and it never behaves as a sociable sheep—a matter which is of some concern to sheep-farmers (Scott) (25).

It is, of course, easy to laugh off these examples from the animal world and to insist that human beings are very different. It is none the less striking to find such similar points of view developing between ethologists and psychoanalysts, and that it is particularly in the field of love relationships, their growth in time and their development within the organism, that the psychology of human beings seems to show the most obvious signs of our animal inheritance.

How can a human infant's experiences affect his or her later relationships and mental health? The principal *sequelae* of separation are threefold: increased anxiety and dependency, increased hatred for the mother, and a tendency to turn away altogether from love objects. This extreme result of separation was one of the first to be noticed and was found among those affectionless characters who cannot give their hearts to anyone, because they have suffered too much pain in their early years (Bowlby) (2). We know now that the affectionless character is not the most frequent result of prolonged separation, for only a minority of children who suffer separation develop this particular character. Even so, if a child has the experience of first giving his affection to one mother figure and that relationship is ruptured, and then to another and that is ruptured, after four or five times the majority of children probably develop a more or less affectionless character.

We have been particularly interested in the process by which the child develops into an affectionless character—unable to make an affectionate relationship, even with an opportunity to do so. There are many instances of affectionless characters among those who never had an opportunity for their affection to flower at a critical period in their infancy. Goldfarb (14) in particular, studied children who had been brought up in a bad institution for the first three years of their life, where they had had no opportunity to make relationships.

A much commoner experience, however, is that of the child who, having built up a love relationship with his mother figure in his first six or twelve months of life, has it shattered. Variations among children are considerable, but practically all children by the age of 12 months have made a highly discriminated love relationship. Some children have made it by 5 or 6 months. Once made, this relationship can be broken. In the film *A Two Year Old Goes to Hospital*[1] it was broken for eight days. One of the most interesting features of that film is the child's inability to greet her mother when she visits her. When the mother appears *Laura* cries and remains lying down. One might have supposed that after crying for hours for her mother

---

[1] *A Two-Year-Old Goes to Hospital.* See p. 123 and Film List, p. 297.

she would rush into her mother's arms; but instead of that she withdraws and turns away (Bowlby *et al.*) (3).

Again, when her mother leaves her, *Laura* just sinks into herself. Though she does not show much open hostility towards her mother, it was noticeable that the doll which was given her in hospital was never treated with kindness and was sometimes treated brutally. But some children, after brief separation, are extremely hostile to their mothers. One small boy, on returning home from hospital, bit his mother's hand until it bled. Moreover, children who are in hospital for a long time commonly destroy the toys which are brought them by their parents. Such hostility can be a very serious psychiatric symptom. Another symptom is the child's rejection of substitute figures, as shown by *Laura* who was uninterested in the nurse.

These phenomena illustrate the earliest stages of a disorder in object relationships. A study of fifty children aged between 12 months and 4 years, separated from their parents, showed that the great majority of them fretted. This fretting can go on for varying lengths of time; one little girl fretted for seventeen days. We have called this phase that of Protest (Robertson) (24). It seems probable that the better the relationship between the child and his mother the longer is the protest: the notion that it is only the spoiled or the neurotic child who frets is certainly mistaken. But after a time every child will give up, for no child can fret or protest indefinitely.

After a few weeks a phase develops which we have described as Denial.[1] The children seem to become happy and settled, even 'hail fellow well met' with the staff. But they have no love object, no one person means more to them than another. Their relations with their mother are clearly impaired, so that it is sometimes said that the child has forgotten his mother. This would be a very serious thing and nothing to be pleased about, because it means that his relation with his love object has been gravely disturbed. In terms of psycho-pathology, we can observe a repression in the course of development—the repression of dependency on and feeling for the mother. Mothers are very sensitive to this change in the child's relationship with them.

What responses occur when the child returns to his mother? Commonly a child on returning home is manifestly upset. Sometimes he is quite unable to respond emotionally, and for a time may behave like an automaton or a doll—in a good, conforming, un-childlike way. But returning feelings and resumed relationships may be stormy; he becomes clinging, demanding and jealous.

[1] *It seems probable that a more accurate term to describe this phase is Repression since the child's feelings towards his mother are repressed.*

A child, on return may not even recognize his mother. Five months after the film record, during her mother's confinement, *Laura* was away in the care of her grandmother for five weeks without seeing either of her parents. When the mother at last returned home, she spoke to *Laura* on the telephone and *Laura* was excited and eager, but when she actually got back home and looked at her mother, she became completely blank and said 'But I want my Mummy'. For forty-eight hours she behaved as though she had completely lost her memory of her mother. She recognized her father and everything else in the house. Events such as this are by no means uncommon.

Hatred towards their mothers is a common feeling of children on their return: they punish their mothers, and older children, particularly, are apt to be accusatory towards them.

It is hardly surprising that someone with intense ambivalence towards a loved object will prove later in life to be a bad spouse and an unsatisfactory parent. Problem parents not infrequently have had periods of deprivation in their own childhood. For instance, there was a case of a maladjusted child whose parents, educated and decent people, were on bad terms with each other. During a joint interview, the father was in a mood to deny his problems, but his wife said that she thought the father's problems sprang from the time when he himself was in hospital, at 5 years old, with suspected tuberculosis. This led the father to recount his story. He had been looked after by a woman doctor towards whom he had developed violent feelings of hatred. During his five months in hospital, his mother had visited only once and he was so angered that when she sent him toys he systematically broke them up. He had felt 'If she can't come herself I don't want her toys.' It appeared that this boy, when he developed into manhood, had never been able to trust women, and even at this interview he went into a long diatribe about women's shortcomings. This attitude had naturally affected his marriage relationship.

Another case is that of the mother of a boy of 11 who would not go to school. The truth is that his mother would not let him go, though this was not overt and conscious on her part. The mother had been brought up in an institution and described this boy as the first thing she had ever had to love in her life.

Why do these experiences have worse effects on some people than on others? It is not unlikely that heredity plays a part in respect of the capacity of individuals to make relationship with their love object. Not only may different children of the same chronological age be at quite different stages of development, but some children appear to be more sensitive to these experiences than others. These possibilities will have to be studied.

Theories of learning in psychology are mostly concerned with learning by normal adults in conditions of no particular stress; but psychiatry is frequently concerned with learning by immature individuals under conditions of intense stress, defining stress as that which is experienced by a highly motivated organism in a problem situation where a solution is either impossible or very difficult. Experimental psychology suggests that responses learned under stress are very resistant to erasure, and those learnt by the immature organism may also have this property.

In the practical field of preventive mental health, separation studies have already proved of value since, once the dangers of separation are appreciated, many social practices are seen to be in need of reform. In the theoretical field not only do they seem to throw light on the development of early object relations but they may provide a focus for the integration of different approaches to the study of personality and its disturbances, including those of psychoanalysis; experimental psychology with animals; learning theory; instinct theory derived from animal psychology; and, finally, genetics.

DISCUSSION

So far there appears to be no evidence of a connection between the degree of intensity and the duration of the protest period, on the one hand, and any such factor as temperament or the degree of activity or inactivity displayed by the children as young babies, though such a connection is, of course, possible.

Where there is acute distress in the child, there may well be a parallel anxiety and distress on the part of the mother, and a certain amount of communication may occur.

In discussing whether the sharing of the care of the child among neighbours or relatives can be a preventive against the effects of such a separation, the attitude of the mother must be taken into account, perhaps regardless of other people, including even the father. The child reared in a large family is, on the whole, much less afraid of strangers than the only child.

The corresponding attitude of the mother towards the child has so far been neglected by psychiatrists. If mothers are to be good mothers their motherhood must be treated with some respect and understanding. It is certainly probable that if the child protests at separation for a long time, the mother is protesting also.

Hospital almoners also have their difficulties in understanding this problem. Nowadays, treatment of children's diseases is so much more effective that children need not spend so much time in hospital. It is far from certain that, with young children, convalescence, meaning a further separation from the mother, is necessary or advisable.

'A TWO-YEAR-OLD GOES TO HOSPITAL'

John Bowlby and
James Robertson

MR. ROBERTSON presented a film entitled *A Two-Year-Old Goes to Hospital*.[1]

In the course of discussion, Dr. Bowlby said: Mr. Robertson and I have been engaged in research into the effects on personality development of separation from the mother in early childhood. During the last four years we have studied three questions: (i) what effect, if any, did these separations have? (ii) what processes do these effects go through? and (iii) in so far as there are bad effects, what do we do about it?

The general proposition that separation in the early years of life can have permanent adverse effects now belongs to history. How these effects come about is something of which we know less. This film shows the behaviour of the child in hospital during eight days of separation from its parents.

Mr. James Robertson said: Starting with the preconception that the child of about 2 years is very dependent upon his mother for security and comfort, I was struck by the undercurrent of unhappiness in children's hospital wards, even in wards which at first sight seemed bright and cheerful. The staffs of the institutions seemed to be little aware of this, as if they were blinded to the unhappiness of these young children. It seemed that two things were happening: first, the system of nursing is such that the care of young children is commonly shared by so many people that no one has a continuous impression of a child, and secondly, and more important, the unhappiness of very young children is so painful that the staffs were turning a very blind eye to it. There seems to be a kind of 'two-way conspiracy': the staff tends to deny this unhappiness, but the children, after a day or two of gross misery, also make an attempt to be quiet and 'good'.

DISCUSSION

What can be done in the home by the parents to ameliorate the effects of separation? Could, for example, neighbours help to share

[1] See Film List, p. 297.

the responsibility? Are things easier in families with several siblings, or the mother out at work?

The behaviour of the child in the film seemed to be quite incredibly good, though her façade occasionally cracked, to reveal underlying misery. Older children can become truly 'settled' because of their greater maturity and ability to understand.

It would be an improvement in hospital procedure, however, if the child were not plunged into the bath immediately on admission, but only after the child had become, to some extent, adjusted; also to allow the mother to put her child into her cot at first and to remain for three or four hours.

In a 'work assignment' system, all the nurses share all duties. In one well-known and reputable hospital thirty-three nurses had something to do with a child who was in there for fifteen days; an experience which is quite frightening for a very young child. A better system of nursing for young children is that of the 'case assignment', in which a nurse looks after a particular child.

It is probable that if people were aware of the emotional signifi-cance of separation experiences, the number of children who are made unhappy could be greatly reduced. For example, need a child be taken into hospital? May it not cost much less to provide, at its own home, medical and surgical care, and nursing assistance for the mother?

It is sometimes proposed that there should be no visiting of child-ren in hospital by their parents 'in order to avoid repeated distress'. There is no evidence to suggest that infrequent visiting would lessen the amount of distress to the child. Young children do not under-stand why they have lost their mother's care, and to be left unvisited in hospital must seem like being abandoned. Frequent visiting may evoke tears, but it allows angry feelings to be expressed and keeps alive some idea that the mother has not completely abandoned the child. But perhaps even frequent visiting is not adequate for the needs of the young child; it may be that only the care of the mother and/or one substitute will suffice.

The behaviour of the child on leaving hospital deserves mention. Most young children are emotionally upset on returning home; and one way in which they show it is by not recognizing their mothers at first, to the great distress of the latter, and later becoming extremely dependent and babyish, aggressive and regressive and so on.

'THE CASE OF MONIQUE'

Jenny Aubry

IN OUR RESEARCH we have studied separation of children from their mothers from the age of 1 year to 3 years old. The initial reaction is approximately the same for every child of less than 3 years of age: first, a phase of acute distress—it cries, calls for its mother, protests, is very upset, is inconsolable, and weeps. This stage of acute distress, which can have serious consequences, including a genuine state of shock, continues for from one to three weeks, after which the child gives some appearance of having adapted itself to its new situation. Close observation will show that this is not a real adaptation but rather that the child no longer has the strength to struggle, and gives up, although he continues to suffer. If the child is approached at that time, he may cling to the person who approaches him and then begin to weep and cry again. Then, after the separation has lasted more than several weeks or months, little by little the child not only ceases to demand any form of motherly care but may even reject the care which is offered. His state at that time is one of apathy and distress, and introverted lack of interest in the exterior world. During this last period the child becomes incapacitated in his ability to establish relations with other children and adults, and it seems that this incapacity leaves an indelible mark on the subsequent formation of his personality.

The first part of the film, *Monique*,[1] shows something of the group life which the children are living. There are individual toys, air, space, room, light, nurses, and kindergarten swings, chutes and all the playground material; but in spite of all these, the life of the children is not very active. They are solitary and their movements are, so to speak, restricted. Among them it is possible to observe some of the typical aspects of a progressive degradation of the personality and loss of contact with the exterior world. I would add that none of these children has any organic illness; their diet is adequate; and, in spite of appearances, they have no disorders of the nervous system.

The film shows the typical behaviour of these children who have been separated from their mothers for more than five months with practically no substitute for maternal care; and they have, in addition, undergone a number of changes by transfer from one hospital to another, for various reasons.

[1] See Film List, p. 297.

125

The film also shows one of these children in the course of the healing process, that is to say, during the course of psychotherapy, which continued for two years. This girl's case has been described under the name of *Monique*.[1]

Monique came to us at the age of 2 years and 2 months; she had been separated from her mother at the age of 3 months and had undergone nine changes of care. The mother had been separated from her child because of insanity, and *Monique* had been sent to us for observation, in order to decide whether the trouble was hereditary or whether it was psychogenic, and if there was anything that we could do for her. In spite of *Monique*'s condition, and after a very long period of observation, we decided that perhaps her state was not constitutional. When we tried to establish contact with her, *Monique* seemed to withdraw into herself and shrink from that contact; but after a few very brief contacts which had lasted only a fraction of a second, we had noticed that a light appeared in her eyes and she seemed to become vivacious for a very short time, after which she again relapsed into her habitual apathy, or had a fit of anxious despair.

We therefore tried to institute a form of treatment, and as soon as she established a relationship with the therapist her attitude to her background and to objects began to change. In particular, she had a very special attitude towards her food: throughout the period during which she refused any stable and permanent relationship with an adult, she had the same hesitation in her relationship to food, and particularly to milk and her bottle; and it was at the moment when she allowed herself to relax in the arms of Genevieve Appell that she could also accept the bottle. For a long time she was divided between her desire for maternal care and the fear which she had of receiving it.

Monique has carried on with her treatment, and later was taken by one of her aunts and is now leading a more or less normal life in a more or less normal family background. There are, of course, some ways in which she is not quite perfect, but we hope to be able to follow up the case and see the result of this treatment at a later date.

Some of these children have perhaps been treated successfully, but at what cost! Is it possible to prevent children from getting into this condition? Would it not be better not to have to treat them? *Monique* took up some 350 to 400 sessions of one hour each, before we were able to put her back into a normal family background; that was a very long, costly and difficult proceeding, and one wonders what measures could have been taken to have prevented

[1] A case studied at the Seminar, but not included in Vol. II.

her from getting into this condition. Not only have children like her been separated very early from their mothers, but in addition there have been no substitutes for maternal care, or very few, and such children have suffered a great number of changes; so that even if no more than a mediocre institution had found somebody permanent to look after them or give them substitute care, these changes of placing would have made it impossible to give them the conditions they needed.

The changes have been due in part to the nature of institutional life, when because of epidemics and contagious diseases contracted there, the children have had to be transferred to a measles ward, or a chicken-pox ward, and then have been sent on to another institution, thereby making the damage even greater.

We must also consider to what extent maternal care might have been sufficient to do the work of this prolonged psychotherapy. Sometimes maternal care and a good family background are enough to bring about recovery, but not always. *Monique* had been placed twice for five months, each time with a good foster-mother who had brought up other children with no difficulty, but who found it impossible with *Monique*. With her, as with others, there was the need for something else, and psychotherapy facilitated a recovery which would not have been possible in the average family background. This is a very important conclusion, because the number of children whom one therapist can take for treatment is limited and selection is a vital issue. We have now seven under treatment and about thirteen who have been treated; and when we make a decision to begin psychotherapy with one, that blocks the chances of another child. Thus we must also try to evaluate the possibilities of recovery without psychotherapy, since that is much easier. During observation over a period of two to three weeks, a number of tests or examinations are made and the child is put in situations where one tries to establish relationship and to evaluate his capacity for receiving from and giving to an adult. If this capacity appears to be sufficient the child is placed in a family, under good conditions, in an attempt to avoid recourse to long-term psychotherapy.

DISCUSSION

At first, *Monique*'s Developmental Quotient could not be assessed because she refused almost every activity. Any attempt to get in touch with her produced more withdrawal. At a second attempt her Developmental Quotient was 40, and at the third it was 110, showing a gain of 70 points.

Natural growth during a year and a half does not explain her development, and this can be illustrated by the way she learnt to walk. *Monique* could not walk at the beginning of the treatment but eventually she learnt to walk within a period of fifteen days. Though she had all the motor equipment for walking she did not use it. She had been stationary for a very long time and had even regressed although she had been placed for five months with a good nurse.

Should one go ahead at once with placing the child in a family, while at the same time beginning psychotherapy? Dr. Aubry said that normally the child was placed in a family only when he had reached a certain degree of development and maturity. Earlier placement might be ideal, but present conditions practically forbid the placing of children in Paris itself; and placement in a rural district cannot be combined with treatment. But in any case, children who do not respond in any way to the affection offered them are difficult propositions for nurses and even more for foster-mothers, who react very badly if the child refuses affection and cries whenever they try to be nice to him.

In the course of psychotherapy the therapist's part is in some respects maternal, but it involves many other responsibilities. At first the child establishes a relationship only with the therapist, but once established, a mother-substitute must be found for the child who is now capable of accepting affection from another person. At such a moment a nurse, as it were, adopted *Monique*. That meant that she could be placed in a family, provided that the treatment be continued (since her food, toilet habits, and so on were still abnormal, and separation from the therapist, if too rapid and sudden, might lead to severe consequences.)

A conspicuous absentee from this group of very subdued, damaged children, is the child to whom, at a slightly older age, the nurses will refer as a 'run-about'. These children in early infancy show ceaseless activity, they learn to walk at roughly the normal time; they are very interested in things but do not differentiate between things and persons. When their attention can be held sufficiently long for a test, their intellectual and motor development is sometimes found normal. They remain very lively but very unapproachable.

Their absence from this group may be because this may be a phenomenon of children separated from their mothers at a much later age, after being able to walk. They also tend to be intolerable in the group, and foundling institutions will not tolerate such children, so they gravitate to mental deficiency colonies at a very early age.

Generally speaking, but not in the case of *Monique,* as the children recover there is a period when they become extremely aggressive, very agitated and may try to run away. If there are more than three children in this stage, at the same time, in the group, the strain on the nurses is too great. The aggressiveness of the children is so intolerable, or they run away to such an extent that either the children have to be restrained, or the nurses refuse to continue to look after them. Hence care has to be taken to space out treatments.

The conclusion is becoming more and more widespread that the problem of young children separated from their mothers is not soluble in institutions unless the latter are organized to reproduce the structure of the family: that is to say, little houses for not more than eight to ten children, all of different ages, in the care of a house-mother and a house-father. Where there is a collective life for the children, or where a nurse has ten children of less than 2 years of age to look after, a substitute mother on a permanent basis cannot be found, if only because of the time off-duty of the personnel. Only a nurse on duty twenty-four hours a day and 365 days a year can do the job required. Even a bad mother is there all the time.

A child who has been separated from his own mother and given to a foster-mother or to an institution which reproduces a normal family, may avoid the unfortunate consequences seen in the film of *Monique*, provided that there is not more than one change. A child often suffers a second change with less facility.

There is also danger to the child in the use of an institution for purposes of observation, before placing him definitely in a family.

As an alternative, in the U.S.A., for instance, there are women who receive a small retaining fee to be available, in urgent cases, to receive children on the same day that they are needed. While they look after the child they are paid as a foster-mother, and then revert to a permanent retaining fee, to be always available. It is not absolutely essential to place the child first in an institution.

The stereotyped movements of abandoned children show a great similarity with the movements seen in a group of schizophrenic patients, but tend to disappear during the course of treatment.

Rocking exists in various forms: nearly always children in institutions will rock for, say, an hour a day. When they are bored, tired or upset they will rock for about five minutes; and if something comes along to arouse their interest, they stop. This gentle, discontinuous rocking appears to be a sign of a search for satisfaction within the child's own person. If a child rocks, it is affording itself some pleasure and a certain isolation from the outside world. Out of twelve hours consciousness a day, some damaged children will rock for ten hours.

In some respects the various manifestations sometimes observed in these children fit into a framework of extra-pyramidal motility, such as lack of co-ordination in movements of the different segments of the fingers, and rigidity of the face. The level of disintegration in these children is a very complex psychomotor problem. The evidence does not point to a definitive lesion in the nervous system.

In a certain number of cases there are modifications of the electro-encephalogram, particularly in those children with very abnormal motility, who sometimes cut themselves off completely from the outside world, with or without rocking, and nearly always with gestures which are quite peculiar, such as putting objects very close to their eyes. Moreover, an organically backward child can undergo a separation trauma, and when the two clinical pictures are super-imposed their differentiation is very difficult.

GROUP INFLUENCE
ON PERSONALITY DEVELOPMENT

Juliette Favez-Boutonier

IN DISCUSSING the influence of social relations on the behaviour of young children, I shall refer throughout to those children living almost entirely in a group of children of the same age, so that we must consider, first, the psychology of the child of from one or two years of age.

That these children have a feeling for their fellows, a reaching out towards them, is shown by their spontaneous interest and curiosity; but I do not know whether any information exists about the conditions in which this interest develops. Dr. Spitz has shown at what age the child notices the human face, but I do not know of any comparable study as to the age at which, or in what circumstances, children pay particular attention to other children of their own age. My own observations suggest that this happens between the first and second year, and it seems probable that it follows the baby's discovery of his own image. The child takes an interest in creatures like himself once he has begun to take an interest in his own self. Children under one year, for instance, show no sign of identifying themselves with a group, but as soon as they begin to walk and so become a bit independent, you will see them trying to mix with other children, to touch them and put their arms around them. I saw, by chance, in the Metro in Paris, two mothers, each with a toddler about 18 months old, whom they had placed on the floor; and although the mothers were not speaking to each other, the children were feeling each other's faces and petting each other, as though there were a kind of spontaneous sympathy between them.

The film, *A Backward Look at Abbey's First Two Years*,[1] has a scene which shows how very young children behave in a group. Abbey and the other children are just over a year old: they are sitting very close to each other with an air of slight embarrassment, as though they do not quite know what to do. They touch each other, but the general impression is that the child making this approach is treating the other as an accessory, or an extension of his own person. He caresses the other, but he might equally well pull his hair or stick a finger in his eye. He will give him something that he is holding

[1] See Film List, p. 297.

131

himself, but will take it back immediately. It is as though he were confused between his own personality and that of the other child. Though this interplay may look very appealing to spectators, it shows, in reality, a lack of differentiation rather than the existence of social consciousness.

The best examples I know of relationships between children, are those described by Anna Freud and Dorothy Burlingham in *Infants Without Families* (5). These authors, for example, describe the case of Rose, aged 21 months, who being still hungry after she has eaten her first plateful of food, cries 'More, more!' The nurse, sitting near Rose, feeding Christopher aged 16 months, gets up to give Rose a second helping. Rose then seizes Christopher's spoon, still crying 'More!' as though she were going to eat his food; but, instead, she feeds Christopher, as though her own wish to eat, and the feeding of Christopher, were confused in her mind.

Another example is that of Stella, aged 18 months, and the 15-months old Agnes. Stella takes Agnes's spoon to try and feed her, but instead, puts the spoon into her own mouth. This is the opposite of the previous example; she starts out to feed Agnes but proceeds to feed herself. Next she puts the spoon into Agnes's mouth, but now the spoon is empty. She does this several times, and finally pours the food on Agnes's plate into her own. So, having started by wanting to feed Agnes, she finishes by feeding herself. This again is a type of confusion of the other person with oneself.

The first point to consider, then, is that of a simple identification, or a sort of sharing in the life of another, on the level of mutual aid and generosity. But there is another aspect which is sometimes even more striking, that of the aggressive reaction, which is just as spontaneous and as frequent as the sympathetic. When the child is hindered in his efforts or frustrated in his desires by some other child, he will oppose him with all his might; it is almost as though he cannot bear that the other child should be different from him. He himself wants to be like the other, or to be close to him, in a way that leads to a confusion of identity; but as soon as he comes up against the reality of the difference between himself and the other, he becomes aggressive. We all know that young children of this age cannot play long together; they quarrel over toys and fight, and very soon adults have to intervene. The aggressive reactions between children of this age are very marked: they bite and pinch each other without restraint, they pull each others' hair, hit each other over the head with whatever they have in their hands, and knock each other over. All this is done, usually, without any apparent awareness of the harm they are doing; but if they are made to realize it, they seem to be pleased with the harmful results. If one says to a child of this age 'You have hurt the other child', very often, instead of looking upset or sorry, he starts all over again as if, now that he knows he is hurting the other one, his only desire is to do it again. Sometimes we may see a shadow of regret later on, but that is usually because the adult has become angry at his behaviour. Then sometimes the child may manage to look sorry.

The spontaneous appearance of aggression is also striking. Anna Freud describes some typical cases, such as, when two children are fighting over a toy, the others who have nothing to do with the quarrel join in and hit either child. Aggression is contagious, as it were; they join in the fight quite spontaneously, as though there were some aggressive stimulus which had affected them, and aggressiveness, at this age, does not appear to be under control any more than is sympathy.

What educative value can there be in such contacts between children of this age? Anna Freud describes, in *Children in Wartime* (6), the first normal reaction as being that of submission to strength. Some children are stronger than others, and those who are strongest, most active, or aggressive, set out to impose their will on the others. After a time, in a group, there will always be some children whom the others dare not attack, or whom they respect, because they are afraid of them. This respect of strength, this ascendancy of might, is a sort of education, though a primitive one.

Children who are more intelligent, more active, or more successful in what they undertake, also gain a kind of ascendancy, due to the admiration that they inspire in the rest. They, also, succeed in dominating others. It can be seen, therefore, in small groups of children at all events, that elements essential for adaptation to social life are learnt by the experience of being in such groups. The children learn to control their aggressiveness because of the reaction which they come to expect, and they learn to discriminate between their desire and its realization. In this way a form of social adjustment emerges which is comparable to real education, and it is possible for a social relationship, even a disciplined society, to exist among children at this age. But, on reflection, it will be seen that the stronger children do not come under the discipline of such a society, which, if it is educational for those who have to submit to those stronger than themselves, is less so for those who impose their will. Seen from this angle, a process of social adjustment of this kind appears to be more like training than education; and there is, to my mind, a great difference between the two.

The result of training, as distinct from education, is that it causes the individual to give up a certain form of behaviour, but no more than that. Something is forbidden; the child acquires a new behaviour but nothing more. Education, on the other hand, attempts to help the child to acquire new capabilities, without limiting his behaviour. There is a vast difference between the two. One can say that an animal is trained, but not that he is educated; for if the animal is well trained he will do what he has been taught to do, but the training has limited and determined his behaviour. For an animal without an inventive mind this does not matter; but for a child with a natural bent for creating new behaviour patterns, training must be more unproductive than education. Through education a new attitude of mind, a new understanding, make possible the development of new and different forms of behaviour.

To make another comparison, the kind of society created by these groups of small children, is comparable to those primitive societies in which 'might is right', such as packs of animals or some adolescent gangs. These phenomena are doubtless human, but not of a high order of humanity. The gang is usually under the tyranny of a bully, the leader or chief, who dominates by reason of his strength and aggressiveness. The rest are forced to submit to his will, and become his instruments or his playthings. This 'boss' type is not a very likeable creature in the social order, and the gang or herd is the most rudimentary form of social organization.

These children's groups, then, do not seem to be of much value educationally as, from the psychological point of view, they are not productive. If adults do not intervene to help such a group to develop, the children will continue to live a life below their own optimum level. If fifteen or twenty children of between 1 and 2 years of age were not looked after by an adult, with regard to their material needs, they would die of privation, and it seems to me that in the psychological sphere the same thing applies. We do not realize sufficiently that, though materially such groups may neither be neglected nor abandoned, they are sometimes severely deprived in the social and psychological sense. This is the main problem of institutional life. When children of 1 or 2 years old live a communal life under conditions in which they are left to themselves all day long, and adults only intervene in order to give them meals or other material care, there results a deficiency, a lack of contact with the adults, that is sufficiently serious to leave a lasting mark upon the personality of the children.

It has been demonstrated that children who have lived in societies deprived of the presence of an adult with a parental role, show an intellectual backwardness that is sometimes so severe as to make them appear to be mentally defective. An example of this is the case of *Monique*.[1] The link which *Monique* established with the adult in

[1] See p. 125.

the course of psychotherapy enabled her to recover and to regain capacities which appeared to be lost; but many children, who have been deprived of close and constant contact with an adult, are not able to take part in normal social life when they are taken from the institutions in which they have been limited in their companionship to children of their own age. The best analogy of the outcome of such a situation is that if the children were really left to themselves, they would die mentally, just as they would die physically if their material wants were not supplied.

It is, of course, adults with whom the children must be able to form adequate ties. As Anna Freud has pointed out, if children living in a residential nursery school can be organized in groups of four or five around a grown-up with a mother role, whom they may call 'mummy', they will accept her straight away. It is very striking that wherever this has been tried, there has been the same result: the children spontaneously attach themselves to her and accept, as if they had been impatiently awaiting her, someone who becomes, as it were, their mother. This pseudo-mother can engender violent feelings of attachment and will cause strong emotions in that children's society, to such an extent that, at first, the presence of this mother may appear to have results which are more troublesome than helpful. The children become more violent, jealous, and aggressive among themselves than before, but now their behaviour is in relation to an adult, and appears to be a normal phenomenon. It is more normal to have feelings than not to have them; and, moreover, their aggression seems to be more easily controlled when there is a sort of system of reference to an adult, for when they give up their aggression it will be for a reason, not for nothing. For instance, the child who is not able to take a toy from another because the other is strong enough to hang on to it, may derive some training from the episode, but he is also utterly frustrated—he has not got the toy, and he has not got anything else. But if he is with someone who is in the relationship of a mother to him when this happens, and she explains the situation to him, there will be some compensation for his frustration, at least in the interest aroused in the mother. Even if he does not understand the explanation there will still remain the fact of her interest to help him to bear his frustration, and he will have received something in exchange. Of course, she may only scold him, but even that may be better than nothing.

The mother, then, is an essential need of children of this age, although this need may be less obvious than that of the suckling baby. To children of the age of 1 or 2, the mother is still a great good, of which they should not be deprived. If she is not there the child is deprived, not only by her absence, but of other things to which a mother's presence would have given some value. The 'reference system' to the adult, as I have called it—the adult who judges, rejects, accepts or intervenes in the children's relationships with each other—gives these relationships a different value and a social significance which they would not otherwise have had.

No social life is possible without the acceptance of certain frustrations, and it cannot be said that frustration itself is always harmful. For example, a child who is prevented from doing what he wants to do may react in two different ways: he may show a reaction of adjustment and make an effort in some other direction, using his intelligence and personal resources to find new or different solutions to his difficulties. Such a reaction is essentially progressive and socially constructive, and leads to integration into society and tolerance of frustration. Secondly, there are maladjusted reactions, in which the frustrated subject, instead of trying to overcome his difficulties, may either turn in upon himself and retreat into autistic behaviour in search of regressive satisfaction; or become aggressive, refuse to tolerate his frustration and attack the person who is the cause of it. Reactions such as these are socially destructive.

Have we any means of knowing *when* frustration will produce favourable or unfavourable results? There are limits beyond which children, depending on their age and capacity, cannot bear frustration, but there seems as yet to be no method of determining this limit exactly. It is important, however, to remember that the mother is the child's most valuable possession and that if he has no mother he starts by being deeply frustrated by this lack, so that all additional frustrations will carry for him the added risk of bringing asocial reactions in their train.

This is the explanation of the phenomena described by the team working under Dr. Aubry in a nursery school belonging to an Institution. The nursery school teacher said that her training had not prepared her to meet with such aggressive, asocial, greedy, and generally troublesome children; but this is understandable if one remembers that these children were fundamentally frustrated in that they had no mother. To the child who has a mother, it is sufficient that he knows that she exists: the fact that she is normally the person who looks after him, and that he knows he can refer to her, gives him a feeling of security which helps him to stand up to his difficulties.

I had an experience, which illustrates this, with a child of under two years of age, who was just beginning to walk well, and who, on his first day in the country, fell head-first into a stream. A little later, I heard him come out of the house, walk a few yards, and then call 'Mummy, Mummy!' His mother was in the house and, not being able to hear him, did not answer. Then he said to himself out loud, 'Mummy is there, Mummy is there', and took a few more steps. This happened several times while he continued his walk. By evoking his mother's presence in this way he was giving himself courage to meet whatever might happen to him.

The mother's role is still an active one even if she is not actually there, and there is a phase in the social adaptation of a child in which not only the mother but every member of the family counts. For the children studied by Anna Freud the absence of the father also made itself felt; but this is still more important after the age of 2 years.

I shall conclude by referring to the important psychological phenomenon which psychoanalysts have termed the Oedipus complex. I think that, in our civilization, the Oedipus complex represents something of capital importance in the life of the child, because it is the symbol of his acceptance of certain frustrations in order to reach higher values. Psychoanalysts have often discussed whether societies can exist with or without the Oedipus complex. It has been said, for instance, that in a non-patriarchal society there may be no Oedipus complex, since the latter is the outcome of a certain attitude towards the father. This may be true, but the fact remains that at a certain stage the child must learn not to think of the family as something belonging to himself alone. He must become aware of the need to share his family with its other members, to allow the mother to belong to the father, and vice versa. Thus there is a close link between the Oedipus complex and the general law of prohibition of incest in human society, the universal existence of which is indisputable.

It has been pointed out, and in my opinion this is extremely important, that although no biological principles are contravened by incest, all human societies prohibit it. It is the only cultural law that is universal. The prohibition means that the child who has attached himself to his mother and has seen in her his first love object and the person who has helped him to accept certain frustrations, must next agree to be frustrated both in and by her, in that he must allow her to belong also to others. This is an essential condition for the formation of human society, which would be impossible if everybody remained attached exclusively to their own parents, and could not form relationships other than those of infancy.

The child is prepared for giving its mother up by the fact that it is not only the mother who counts. There is, at least, the father, and, sometimes, other relations. Even if he is an only child he must eventually agree to share his mother with his father, and if he has brothers and sisters he will have to endure other kinds of frustration.

The problems which arise among children of the same family

137

resemble those that arise in a nursery group, but the fact that in a family each child is of a different age, and that there are bigger or smaller children, constitutes the vital difference between sibling groups in a family and groups in a nursery school. Moreover, the presence and role of parents in the family makes of the latter a group very different from a 'nursery group'. Without parents there cannot arise a situation of the 'Oedipus complex' type; and if this complex is an essential feature of human society, no true society will develop without it.

In my opinion the function of the type of children's society represented by the nursery school, should be limited: it should never be considered as being able to replace, in any way, the family group, but only as a complementary means of apprenticeship to social life. For children of less than 2 years of age, in particular, the nursery group cannot, in any way, be a substitute for the influence of the family on the development of personality.

DISCUSSION

Young Children in Groups. An infants' home in Copenhagen has tried a new method of dividing its forty children into groups, each of which contained, say, a child of from 5 to 6 months old, another from 9 to 11 months, another from 12 to 15 months, and another from 15 months to 2 years of age. They made the room as much like a normal home as possible, and the nurse slept with the children at night.

A move has also been made in nursery schools to put the children into small groups of different ages, with very good results. A number of problems, however, have still to be overcome, such as training the nurses, and the problem of how close the relationship should be between the nurse and the children.

The confusion which the child makes between himself and another child occurs also in relation to parents—a point first made by Susan Isaacs, later followed up by Melanie Klein, and developed in the work of Fairbairn of Edinburgh. According to this theory, the child is unable to distinguish between the 'good' mother who clothes him, feeds him and plays with him, and the 'bad' mother who frustrates him. The child's capacity for aggressive acts is limited, swallowing being the most noteworthy, and if the child incorporates the 'bad' mother within himself only his 'good' mother will remain outside. Fairbairn has suggested that the internal bad mother forms the aggressive part of the personality, which he has termed the 'internal saboteur'. It is thought that the internalization of the internal saboteur takes place about the second or third year. Might not a child in such a stage, meeting another child of its own age, suffer some confusion in his mind as to whether it was the other child or himself who was going through that experience?

The point is very theoretical and it is difficult to prove that when a child is aggressive towards his contemporary he is also aggressive towards an image of the first person who had frustrated him, i.e., his mother. This is a possible concept, but though it may be of practical help in therapy, it is doubtful if it would have practical significance to the life of groups in a nursery. When a child hits a small friend who is not pleasant or who is up against him, it is a manifestation of aggression and, though possibly related to other frustrations in the past, such aggressive manifestations are inevitable. A world cannot be imagined where they do not happen, any more than a child can imagine naturally, that a mother can be good and bad at the same time.

However, such theories may have a practical use in society, particularly among those who misinterpret psychoanalytic doctrine in saying that the great thing is not to frustrate children. Fairbairn holds that the internal saboteur is so severe, frustrating and ruthless that the child welcomes some control of his aggression by an external agency. So that there is a theoretical justification for interfering with crude aggression shown by a child.

The same sort of thing is true of punishment: nothing in the external world can compare in severity with the punishment which an individual is capable of giving himself, and therefore external punishment is often a very comforting thing. Generally speaking, people are too apt to be afraid of exercising control over the crude emotions of children.

Aggression is a considerable problem in nursery schools, and very great difficulties are met with among children deprived of their mothers. Very often toddlers who are frustrated and deprived of maternal care have a kind of aggressive violence which is almost equivalent to self-punishment but at the same time they are in a panic because of the other children's reactions. The child who is too frustrated and has not had the security given by a mother, cannot control his aggressive impulses, whether this be because he did not have a good mother, or has incorporated the bad mother into himself. In practice these are the children who need help: first because when one pays attention to them they stop hitting the others, and secondly, whereas a child knocked about is very soon comforted, the aggressor will continue unless something is done about it. To attend to the aggressive child is not to punish him, but is the best way of protecting them both.

These phenomena might be described more scientifically in relation to the spontaneous reaction of the child to sudden, unexpected events. Strong emotions sometimes produce what Duprez has called emotional anaphyllaxis: in other words the child, in the presence of a new feeling, reacts in an exaggerated and uncontrolled way. On the other hand, emotions sometimes have an educational value which depends chiefly on the circumstances in which they arise. For example, during the war, training was given to soldiers' emotional reactions, as in battle-training schools. If the child, in the presence of other children, reacts in a crude way to emotions caused by human relationships, this is because those emotions are too strong and bring about 'emotional anaphyllaxis'. The parental function in this respect is an educative one, and allows for the control of the emotion.

'Emotional anaphyllaxis' might also be involved in the well-known phenomenon of young children separated from their mothers who, when they do not feel safe, become very aggressive.

The sociological implication of the matter is that on studying different societies in the world it is possible to see that a different kind of character is produced in children in relation to the proportion to which the grandparents, the parents, and children of the same age bring them up. It is possible to suggest that for a strictly tradi-tional society, the grandparents are the most appropriate people to bring up the children, maintaining the style of the past; that in very rapidly-changing societies parents make the best 'bringers-up' of the children; but that when a society is changing too rapidly, it might tend more and more to use age-mates—children of the same age.

The United States of America has moved far towards segregating children of the same age, in ordinary nursery schools. In one of the best nursery schools 'old twos' and 'young twos' are separated and not allowed to be in the same group. All through the school years, and indeed all through American life, there is a tendency to have the child adjust to other children of the same age with as little interven-tion from adults as possible. This produces a different form of identi-fication, a different sense of the self, recently termed a 'radar per-sonality'—one which always pays attention to what the other person is going to do, in order to get a signal for the next item of behaviour. This is related to the behaviour described among the 2-year-olds who have learned not to hit another who would be likely to hit back. Such tendencies have implications not only for institutional care and for the nursery age, but for the whole structure of society.

SPECIAL EXPERIENCES OF YOUNG CHILDREN

PARTICULARLY IN TIMES OF SOCIAL DISTURBANCE

Anna Freud

PART I

ON REFLECTION I can discern four sources of my knowledge about the impact of war-time conditions on the life and development of the child. Early in the World War of 1914–18, we began, in Vienna, to collect children in play groups in order to keep them off the street; and this drew our attention to the impact of the then prevailing war conditions on these children.

The second source of knowledge was a residential institution called the Hampstead Nurseries, opened in London in 1939, which we kept open, with help from an American War Charity[1] until 1945. We saw children here before evacuation or after return as failures of evacuation; and others in our country nursery, where some eighty lived with us more or less throughout the five years of the war.

The third source, after the war, was a small group of child concentration camp victims who had been brought to England as the sole survivors of their families. Five or six of these children were brought up for one year together in Sussex, in a private home under the direction of Miss Sophie Dann (*who was present and joined in the discussion*).

The fourth source was some older concentration camp victims, collected in London in a children's home. Recently I helped the more difficult and abnormal of these children, now adolescent, to find relief for some of their problems and difficulties, in psychoanalytic treatment.

I have certainly concluded that it would be no good to use the knowledge gained about children in one war, for the next; the changes in a future war would be as great as those from the First to the Second World War. The profit from observations of this kind needs to be put to a more indirect use; to the increase of our theoretical knowledge of child psychology, to swell our already existing knowledge of the child.

[1] The Foster Parents' Plan for War Children, Inc.

During a war, our quieter and more profitable methods of learning about children are very rudely interrupted. Schools are dislocated, laboratories are closed, research workers are used for other purposes; but we have learnt a great deal about children during the last two wars.

Those who are concerned with a system of child psychology, which is both dynamic, being concerned with the forces active in the child, and genetic, being concerned with the influence of the child's past on his present development, are handicapped by the lack of opportunity for the type of experiment that academic psychologists find so necessary. Mental life is very complex and not only is it nearly impossible to isolate factors, but to do so in itself distorts the experimental situation. However, in the study of mental conflicts and their outcome, the time-lag between event and consequence may be enormous. No effect may show for a week, a month, a year, five years or even ten years. To establish this empirically would require observation over a period far longer than is usually possible.

Another reason lies in certain properties of human reactions; for the *amount* of the experience is not unrelated to its quality. The loss of a toy is a disappointment, but the loss of the mother shakes the child's whole love life and may even influence, for the future, his ability to form new relationships; the two experiences are not comparable by experimental means.

In war-time, with the enormous upheaval of life, Fate stages something of an experiment, in the sense that it demonstrates the effect of certain factors in the child's life and the consequences of the removal of other factors. For example, so many children lose their fathers or mothers that it constitutes, as it were, an experimental situation which we could never stage ourselves, but which we can watch and find most revealing.

During the war years of 1914 to 1918 two main factors in the children's lives were hunger, or at least lack of proper nourishment, and absence of the father; and for the first time, people began to realize the extent of the difference which that absence makes to the mental development of the child. There was a very noticeable increase in delinquency and an impairment of the smooth social adaptation of these children to group life in schools, to their adolescent occupations, and so on.

Aichhorn, the Viennese youth worker and analyst, author of *Wayward Youth*, studied children of the 1914–18 war who, owing to this partial breaking up of families, lost their social adaptation and became delinquent. During an investigation of the past histories of other young delinquents and criminals, he found that all children of this group had had gaps in their family life very similar to the

142

gaps which were artificially created by the absence of the father during the war. Among them were illegitimate children, children whose father had left the mother early after birth, or who had been handed from one foster-mother to another, and whose moral development had suffered through lack of identification with a steady father figure. That was the important lesson which was learnt from the 'experiments' which the First World War made with children.

On the bodily side, the reduced diet of these children in Europe taught us some very valuable lessons about the aftermath. It is a matter for thought to what degree this experiment led directly to the excellent feeding of the children in England during the 1939–45 war.

Another impressive lesson of the 1914–18 war was that children who have suffered from hunger, especially early in their lives, do not welcome food afterwards but, on the contrary, suffer an estrangement from the pleasures of eating, strong enough to be the basis of disturbances of feeding in later life. After 1918 there was a high incidence, in Vienna, of feeding difficulties in all sections of the population, and I can remember at a parents' meeting—quite a new idea at the time—Aichhorn asked the parents to tell him what was the difficulty in handling their children which came to their minds first. The audience, not used to a discussion, felt shy and embarrassed; after a pause a father got up and said, 'The most difficult thing is to make our little daughter eat her breakfast.' Then a storm broke among the parents and they all described the methods which they used to make their children eat, such as paying a penny for each piece of bread eaten, or promising an outing for each cup of milk drunk.

What about the psychological lessons of the 1939–45 war? In the Hampstead Nurseries there were eighty resident children, from 10 days to 6 or 7 years of age. Some of the children had suffered sudden separations, had had their families broken up; nearly all had absent fathers, and all of them had absent mothers, except for a few whose mothers worked in the nursery.

The effects of separation from the family and from familiar surroundings were both direct and indirect. Infants under 1 year of age reacted directly, almost exclusively with their bodies; with upsets of feeding, sleeping, and digestion, or with slight illnesses such as colds, sore throats, and so on. Their bodies did not function smoothly during separation, and this bodily upheaval was sometimes, but not always, accompanied by an emotional upheaval. We did not understand it at first; we looked for infections, for the wrong ingredients in the food, and tried alterations in the sleeping conditions, until we eventually concluded that these children were reacting to the experience with the body rather than with the mind.

At the next age, mind and body are still in very close relationship but the disturbance shows more on the emotional side. When we took over the care of toddlers from their families, they became not only less smoothly functioning, they also became younger children. This regression showed not only in the child's behaviour but in his whole nature, and in all parts of his life. These children became more dependent, they lost many of the skills which they had already developed; those who had been able to eat alone now had to be fed, those who had been able to fall asleep alone now needed company at bed-time. More impressive, children who had just begun to walk would sometimes give up walking, and those who had just learned their first words or sentences would stop speaking for several weeks and subsequently had to learn to speak afresh. Moreover, and this was also observed on a larger scale in England during the evacuation of children from the towns, those children who had attained bowel and bladder-control in their own homes, lost it.

Many of these very young children had been left by their fathers a short while before; and their evacuation or coming to us meant a final separation from their families. The older children in their families had by then already been evacuated with their schools. I will mention only the two main effects of the breaking-up of the mother-child relationship on the child. First: the child who has lost the really important person in his life does not immediately make a substitute relationship with somebody else, but for a while the child's feeling may be withdrawn from the environment altogether and centred on himself.

Secondly, the feelings which the child previously had for the mother are in need of a substitute object outside himself; but he behaves towards the substitute nurse or nursery worker, or whoever it may be, in a manner appropriate to a much younger child. He displays a more infantile type of love, more demanding, a stomach love instead of real love, a need for sweets and food and care and attention rather than for a relationship with any other person. Moreover, his need is expressed in auto-erotic activities; finger-sucking or other sucking activities with the tongue, lips and mouth, rocking and other rhythmical movements, head knocking, and among older children more masturbation.

Of course, these young infants were offered, as a substitute for their lost families, life in a group of their own age. Though children normally live in groups of their own age in schools, this is quite different from spending their whole life, day and night, in a single-age group which, in the case of nurseries, is composed exclusively of 2, 3, or 4-year-olds. After being for a while in a room where there are eight or ten 2-year-olds one forgets that there is such a thing as

144

speech. Why should one speak? No one else speaks. Children make gestures and understand each other quite well, and if they want something they scream a little, if angry about something, stamp their feet, and everybody understands. It is quite difficult to prevent the adult worker in such a group from forgetting to speak herself; but for whom or from whom else can the children learn to speak?

People were surprised at the aggressiveness of these children of 2 or 2½, but in such a group, everybody is aggressive. The reason is not far to seek: in a family with four or five children, all the older children would get into trouble if they responded to the aggression of the 2-year-old in like measure. The older children are taught to show a great deal of consideration to the aggressive young toddler; but toddlers show no consideration to each other. In a group of toddlers, everybody is unrestrained, everybody is aggressive, everybody grabs toys and no one has the least consideration for anybody else. Instead of overcoming their own aggressive urges, the children are reinforced continuously by the strength of the aggressive urges of the others.

In our experience this leads to very severe sleep disturbances, the children continuing to fight in the night; they talk in their sleep, and say 'No, mine—let go' in the throes of a conflict which has pursued them into the night. Three to five year olds in a group suffer acutely from the monotony of life as well as from the lack of examples set by older children.

We found that children, during the temporary absence of their parents and of any other important adults, form warmer relations with each other than is usual at such ages. They gradually formed companionships, real friendships, and even loves at the early age of 3 and 4. The idea that friendships between children at those early ages would not last longer than the game they were playing at the time, is not true of children living in a group of their own age, some of whom kept up friendships for weeks and months.

Also, in these early age groups a primitive morality develops among the children, different from that which a child acquires in identification with the parents. This primitive morality is based on strength and weakness: not to provoke somebody who is stronger; how to impress somebody who is weaker; not to create too much trouble by grabbing from those who have loud voices and can scream. This leads indirectly to the protection of the weak and also to a primitive form of barter; for instance, one child has a toy engine, and another child who wants it knows that if he grabs that engine, there will be an upheaval and a big scream—so he offers a piece of chocolate or something in exchange. But though such barter represents the beginning of society, might triumphs over right.

L   145

War upheavals also have indirect, far-reaching effects. Children who do not live with their parents, or with satisfactory substitutes, do not make the usual identifications, and so do not develop the usual internal moral agency—the super ego. The super ego may develop incompletely, or with less strength, and so lead later to very serious trouble in social adaptation. Further, children who have experienced no early love life are unprepared for the storms of adolescence.

It is a curious fact that when a child is taken out of his family and put into a nursery group to live, he may need weeks of adaptation to become accustomed to life with other children. On the other hand, we took four children out of our nursery group for adoption in families. One boy of 4 years had come to us at the age of a few months, and had never seen a private family. The second morning when the child was at breakfast with his prospective adoptive parents, the husband got up and kissed his wife goodbye before going to his business. The boy raised a howl; that was his mother and he did not want her interfered with by the father. Thus, after two days, he had learnt something of the psychological set-up of a family. Why should it be so much easier for the child to slip into family life than to slip out of it and get into community life?

Further observations were made of a group of six concentration camp victims (10). All the parents had perished in a Nazi extermination camp and the children had been hidden either by an agency or another family.

These six children had never known their parents; they had been brought up in the concentration camp, in which the Jewish community had evolved a crude sort of self-government. They had lived in very restricted circumstances, in houses in which they were cared for by a few inmates of the concentration camp. They knew nothing of the world, of private life, or of the meaning of 'father' and 'mother'. They had lived ten or twelve to a room which served as bedroom, play-room and eating place; and a yard for exercise, which they shared with other similar houses and which they were not always permitted to use.

Six were about the age of 3 and had come to form a more compact group than the usual homogeneous age group. These six children had all their security in the group and they had no interest in anything in the world outside. They neither had nor wanted to have parents; for quite some time they were not interested in the adults who looked after them, but they were enormously interested in each other. They were so interested in each other's characteristics that they fulfilled each other's wishes and needs just as a mother fulfils the needs of her child. For instance, one of these children wanted

146

to be waited on as if she were a little queen, and so she was served by the others. When a child wanted a special toy in his bed in the evening, one of the others saw to it that the toy was there. When there was food, it was shared out, and when one child received a parcel it was shared with the others; there was no envy and no jealousy. There were no fights, except very occasionally. What impressed me most, however, was that when the children went for walks they carried each other's coats, and bent the branches back in the wood so that the other children could walk through, which I have never seen done among mothered children. The behaviour of these children confirms an idea derived from theoretical formulations that jealousy between brothers and sisters is not a direct envy of what the other possesses but that it is an envy based on their relationship with the parents. The children are jealous of each other, with the figure of the parent in their minds; they are jealous of their competitors for the love of the parent. Where there is no parent, there is group identification instead of sibling rivalry.

We also learnt interesting facts concerning the memory of children. Though the first years of life are blacked out in memory, children usually carry in their minds isolated pictures of the past. These concentration-camp children appeared to have no such pictures of their past; we do not know whether they will bring them up in the future. It seems that when there is no one adult figure accompanying the child through the early childhood years, there is a more complete break with the past than is usual. We carry our recollections of the past with the help of steady relationships which have been continuous through our development; where no such relationships have persisted, it is evidently more difficult to retain early memories.

A further point is that the older concentration camp victims, some of whom have been under psychoanalytical treatment, show a much greater resistance to the revival of their past than is normal at their age. Their past contains so many bad experiences, in some cases of horrors, and in all cases of terrible losses; and though most of them have little of it in their conscious minds, the pressure with which they have to keep closed this chapter of their life is very strong, and it is extremely difficult to break through the barrier.

Naturally, the upbringing of these uprooted and emotionally deprived children presents many difficulties, one of which is that the older among them, near adolescence, have in their minds images of parents of their past which have literally no relation to the real parents. For instance, one child's father, as we learnt by chance, was a small Jewish tailor in the wilds of Poland. But the fragmentary memories of that child depicted a home with all possible comforts and luxuries; nothing that the child was given subsequently could compare with that. Such children have two sets of parents: the substitute parents of later life who, whenever there is conflict, appear to them as bad, depriving and prohibiting, and another set of parents who are ideal. The bad and the ideal sets of parents do not combine, so that the usual mixture of positive and negative feelings of children towards their parents becomes split into positive feelings for the dead parents and negative feelings for their present substitutes. Such a situation becomes especially*difficult in adolescence and when there are no actual parent figures to struggle against. The emotional conflict of adolescence, after all, consists of resolving the parent relationship, positive and negative; but these children have finished with their parent relationship on another basis and long ago.

To sum up: the war should have drawn our attention to our neglect of manifold opportunities for the study of children in peacetime. These deprived children can be found and studied in foundling homes, orphanages and under the effect of hospitalization; day nurseries can show the effects of temporary separation; convalescent homes show temporary separation of longer duration. Other studies of this kind could be suggested; for example, to study in blind, deaf, and crippled children what the senses and the use of the senses contribute to their identifications—the build-up of character and social relationships.

DISCUSSION I

Does psychoanalysis throw any light on whether children remember what happened before adoption? A case is recorded of a child, adopted at 3 years old, who half an hour after being introduced into the house of adoption called his adoptive parents 'father' and 'mother', and a few days later had built up a story that he had previously belonged to those very parents but had been separated from them. On the whole, this question has been neglected in analysis; clinical experience suggests that a child of 3, even if it did not consciously express itself, would know a great deal about its life before adoption.

What should an adopted child be told? One of the concentration camp victims, adopted in America by parents with a very good psychological understanding, had formed a very firm fantasy that he had been born in England. Fairbairn has called attention to the fantasies of children with regard to their parents; of delinquent children at a corrective school who thought their parents were marvellous—rich, powerful, and very kind and loving. One such boy of 14 was always running away and then wanting to return. He had a very firm fantasy that his father was a very important man in his home-town, that his mother was very beautiful and loving, and that they had a well-furnished and comfortable home. All those things were quite untrue, and when he ran away to those wonderful parents and beautiful conditions, he then faced the reality and could not stand it.

Fairbairn postulated that, below the conscious concept of the parents as good, there was an unconscious image of bad, rejecting parents, far worse than the real parents ever were. Herein lay the real conflict. The image of the rejecting, bad, unjust parents was then projected secondarily on to the person who played the parent role with the child.

The evidence of the extent of communication to the child of the attitude of the parent is now being considered. British war-time experience was that frightened mothers communicated directly with very young children. How much can be communicated unwittingly by parents in the event of, for example, adoption and in artificial insemination? It would be interesting to study those day-nurseries where the adults accept that it is right for the children to be there, that they will not quarrel and will gain something from the nursery, as compared with cases where the adults think that nurseries are bad, expect the children to be aggressive, and consider them to be deprived.

How far will an analogy between war and peace and between family children and deprived children respectively, lead more deeply into knowledge of the results of separation between children and parents? First, we need to compare the results of physical separation with the results of those other things which destroy or attack the relationship between children and parents. A problem in personal relations might be cited: a child, whose mother died when the child was 4½, was looked after by a foster-mother for a short time. Later the father married again, and the child was rather a problem when he came back to the father. The foster-mother used to visit them infrequently, and because there were good effects after the visit, it became rather a habit for her to be sent for. On each occasion the crucial point of the visit was that the child would ask a lot of questions, seeking reassurance of how pleasant and nice a person his mother had been. This is an example of a problem which occurs quite often in the ordinary context of relationships and which would appear to be amenable to normal social handling.

What is the effect on children of the partial and recurring separation which occurs in day-nurseries and residential nurseries? At what age will it no longer be dangerous to the child to be taken by the mother in the daytime to a day-nursery and to be left there for many hours? War experience suggests that is extremely difficult for an infant up to 1 year or $1\frac{1}{2}$ years to live under two routines, quite apart from the child's inability to make attachments to two sets of people. The younger the child, the greater the advantage to him to have a minimum of people to look after him and a minimum of outside circumstances to which to adapt. Young children in day-nurseries, though they may have had much better bodily care than at home, suffered from having to adapt to a greater amount and variety of stimulation from outside than they could really manage.

Between the ages of $1\frac{1}{2}$ and $2\frac{1}{2}$ and in a very small group, in very good contact with their parents, and if the nursery hours are not too long, children can benefit in respect of motor development and feeding; and in ego development provided that they are not prevented from moving.

From the ages of $2\frac{1}{2}$ to 3 years and onwards, the only safeguards needed are that the hours should not be too long, the groups not too large, the staff sufficiently knowledgeable, and the child should not be sent there just as a new baby is born.

PART II

Summing up what we know about children's reactions to violent war-time experiences, we could confirm the view that the anxiety of the child is closely connected with the anxiety of the adult with whom he is living; but that violence, as such, does not mean to the child necessarily what it means to the adult. Violence is more natural to the child's mind than to that of the adult, who has taken great trouble to grow out of violence into more moderate forms of living. If the children live with adults to whom destruction, shooting, bombing, and attack are welcome, I think it would all be great fun. However they live with adults who fear the bombs, who are conscious of the danger to their own lives and to the lives of the children, and the children take their cue from the adults. We have to bear in mind that, on the whole, one has to teach the children that these things are bad.

The very young children, of course, do not realize that war is an emergency state and not the ordinary way of life. These children took to bombing as children take to thunderstorms—noisy, disagreeable, frightening, but probably a normal part of life. They slipped into a routine of war living, in itself frightening, with no conception of a peace-time existence. One day the all-clear signal was not given in the early morning. Previously, for some time the bombers had left the sky over London in the early morning and the all-clear signal had been given just in time for everybody to get up. The signal had the significance in the nursery of, say, the dinner-gong; for the children were promptly taken out of the shelter and had their breakfast upstairs. On this particular day the all-clear signal was not given, so the children had to be kept in the shelter, and the adults were, naturally, anxious. One little girl jumped up suddenly and said, 'They have forgotten to switch off the air-raid', just as though the household management was not in order. She could take for granted experiences which meant something horrible to the adults and thus demonstrated a difference between what the child experiences in identification with the adult and his own conception of the matter.

Experience in the occupied and invaded countries, such as Greece, was different. Young children who were hidden with their mothers frequently understood the occupation conditions: for example, a 3-year-old Austrian Jewish girl was hidden with her mother in a Dutch village, with false papers; her mother had impressed on her that she must never say her real name and must never let on to anybody that she was not a real little Dutch girl. The situation was so very dangerous for them that the mother had to threaten the child: 'If you tell our real names, they will take you away from me and you may never see me again.' Evidently the child understood, for during about three years the child never mentioned the matter again, until on the day of the Liberation she said to her mother, 'And can we now have our real name again?'—This is amazing, for it means that the problem was alive in her all the time, but of course, in identification with the mother.

Other war-time experiences for older children and especially boys, have included growing up under conditions of underground life with all its hidden meanings and its secrets to be kept from the occupying forces. The subsequent difficulty has been to bring them back to ordinary drab peace-time morality afterwards. Their attitude was, 'Why not deceive the authorities?'

The most impressive fact about the children who have seen or experienced actual violence—bombing, scenes of death, blood, etc., is that, if the child is not actually shocked in the medical sense, he does not talk about it. Children who had lost their fathers in air-raids, in our experience, did not talk about their loss earlier than about six months to a year later, and I have not seen it come out, even in play, before that lapse of time. Children who had not actually experienced such a thing but only heard about it, used to play at air-raids and would treat them as everyday occurrences.

A boy, who is now 19, who had been through the whole occupation of Holland, and had witnessed killing, the taking away of people and scenes of violence of all kinds, only after six or seven years, began to talk about it. This suggests that the shock, the impact of the experience, has to be worked over before the child is willing to impart it to others.

When mothers and children came to the nursery after air-raids, the children did not mention what had happened, but the mothers talked incessantly, sometimes for days, about their experiences. The adult capacity for verbal abreaction appeared to help the mother to overcome the shock; whereas the child has no such capacity. For the child to talk about it meant danger; for the adult it was a definite relief.

The forcible abduction of children, as, for instance, in Greece, must have made an enormous impression on them, perhaps only mitigated by the fact that they were taken in groups, and at least kept their companions, and maybe their brothers and sisters.

It is horrible if, after children have been deprived of their parents, they are then separated from their siblings, for reasons of administration. To deprive children of the contacts which are still left to them shows such an absolute lack of thinking among those who carry out measures of this kind, that all informed people have a duty to teach administrators what they are doing in that respect. In this connection it was good that these Greek children, after they had been recaptured, were not separated from their brothers and sisters.

Next, we come to the brother-sister relationship. Those who have worked in a residential school, institution, hospital or a convalescent home know that when children from one family arrive and are kept together they act very affectionately towards each other. Under the shock of separation from their parents they do what the concentration camp victims did so intensively: they offer to each other the affection for which they have no other placement at the moment, and they drop the jealousies which have centred around the figures of the parents. Usually this happens for a short time only.

The children would arrive at our nursery after raids on London, two or three together, affectionate little brothers and sisters, putting each other to bed, comforting each other, and very suspicious of all the grown-ups around. But if, after a few days, they had their first quarrel we were very pleased, because it showed that they had begun to feel at home with us. As soon as they made their first transference of feeling to the adults, the old situation of sibling rivalry recurred.

It has been remarked that families may show phenomena according to the quality of the parents' marriage relationship. Where the parents invest most of their feeling in each other and the children are outside that magic circle, sibling rivalry is usually less than in those cases where the parents find no satisfaction in each other, and place their whole affection in the children. It should also be remembered that children learn to quarrel from their parents and practise it on their siblings.

How is the Oedipus complex resolved in children deprived of their homes—a central problem of our study of the Hampstead nursery children? What happens when there is no such situation and there are no Oedipus ties? Among the many things which happen, the most important is the enormous need of the child to construct this situation where it is missing; to give somebody the place of the father and somebody else the place of the mother; to form a three-cornered situation, either with other children or with adults. Such children have a great inner need to use every scrap of information gained from other children who, perhaps, have families and have been visited by them, or who have been home for a short period, to build up a fantasy family of their own. In *Children in Wartime* (6) my colleague, Dorothy Burlingham and I described a few children in this situation, especially one boy who built up a whole father-relationship on the basis of a few visits from his father, who was in the Forces and who did not care much about him. Other children also used items gleaned from here and there to construct these fantasies which are so important for their emotional life.

The exclusively bodily reaction of the child under the age of one really needs careful medical exploration. There seems no doubt that the younger the child, the more is an emotional disturbance likely to be expressed by the body. Many observations made during the analytic treatment of children, of the incidence of colds, stomach upsets, sore throats and similar intercurrent illnesses should have prepared us for this finding. I remember analysing a little boy of 6 or 7 years old, of divorced parents, who lived with his father, and who was passionately attached to his mother. He reacted to every arrival and departure of the mother with a bodily illness. Each time she went away his bodily illness had more than the purpose of keeping her near: it was an expression of the degree of his disturbance, which evidently rendered his body more vulnerable to illness. Many studies have been made of the feeding and sleeping disturbances of children which, we know, are greatly influenced by the emotions, as are constipation and diarrhoea and the regulation of the bowels in general. Such studies should lead further towards the understanding of the role of the body in giving expression to the emotions.

DISCUSSION II

It is appropriate to discuss the general phenomena of violence and danger. A great many adults try to live either in the pre-1914 Golden Age or the pre-1939 Golden Age, which they tend to think of as lush periods of peaceful plenty. They forget such matters as the death-rate on the roads and the suicide rate, and if they were realistic about all the dangers of civilized life, they would realize that in many ways they have always lived in a jungle. It is a different kind of jungle, that is all.

The adult fantasy of the Golden Age really unfits people for realistic thinking about the future. The present state of the world and of scientific invention should lead inevitably to the conclusion that for, say, the next fifty years we must expect to live in a dangerous world.

During the war there had been general surprise at the way children and the civilian population generally, adapted themselves. Most people, and especially the children, had stood up well to those dangerous conditions. Moreover, some people who, before the war, were neurotic and maladjusted and suffering from psychogenic fatigue, had found the experience of air-raids stimulating and had lived a more effective life in war-time. The decline of the suicide rates during both the last two wars also suggested, paradoxically, that many people seemed to find life more worth living in war-time.

A philosophy of civilized life resenting danger as something breaking in on a fantasy of a Golden Age, does not permit clear thinking about the bringing-up of children.

Another illustration is the effect on children of scenes of violence on the cinema screen, but the question of children's adaptation to violence and danger leads to a bigger issue. Young children are violent and do not really mind dangers, but we are carefully taught to recognize dangers and to guard against them. Parents are concerned with a struggle against the child's most important drives, sex and aggression. Do children suppress, repress, or transfer too much of their original drives, so that though they may build up fine character structures, they are hampered, uncertain and unhappy in situations in adult life which call for the full force of the original drive? On the one hand neurosis in adult life is closely connected with repression and transformation of early drives, but on the other hand some people may remain too free in their sexuality and too violent in their aggressive expressions: they are 'a-social' or 'de-social' persons.

With a constant community structure this situation will show only slight shifts from one generation to another: there will be more of the drives left free for dealing with the outside world, or less; more neurosis, or a little less. There is a close inter-relation between these drives and the structure of the adult community into which the child must grow.

The ability of children to talk about experiences of violence depends upon age, i.e., the language and conceptual development of the child, his ability to abstract experiences and to talk about them. The day after an air-raid the whole group of children would play 'air-raid', but only if they had not actually suffered from the air-raid. On the other hand, a child brought in from a bombed house would not play 'bombed house' for, perhaps, six months. The very violence of the experience seems, for the time being, to block the child's way to expression, but the consequences would show in other behaviour: the child would be disturbed or moody, would show loss of appetite, be clinging, would turn away, be extremely noisy; or, coming nearer to expression, be cruel to others. It took a long time before the actual causative happening was brought into expression.

Observations made during the psychological treatment of children may be made years after the event; but in this situation, the full expression comes, if not in words, then in play. One of the reasons why, in the treatment of children, such close contact between the family and the therapist must be maintained, is that there might be important events during treatment about which the child might not talk. The therapist is apt to find out how much more the social worker knows about what is going on than he does himself.

Change of identity has afterwards frequently raised problems of the child's own identification with its name. After the war, a French law allowed all those who, during the war, had taken French names, to retain those names. In some cases this led to further changes, three or four years after the child had gone back to its real identity. Such a child might wonder who it was and what its name really was, and what it would become if it changed names again; and the change was associated, naturally, with very grave difficulties during the war. These problems are well known to analysts dealing with adult patients who have changed names, sometimes, though not always, being associated with a change of religion, notably the Jewish religion, when people make attempts to become assimilated into a new community.

Under some conditions change of name might be thought to be eminently rational, but analytical experience has shown it always signifies some intended abrupt break with the past. Study of peace-time change of name might throw light on change of name under war-time conditions.

With regard to groups of children, another group of concentration camp survivors, somewhat older, were kept together. Their group structure was maintained by their own very severe rules and unbreakable regulations, about sharing food or other advantages. When one of their number broke a rule it seemed to them quite natural to kill him; and they made him jump out of the window. It was apparent that they did not realize, at all, the value normally attached to life.

Various experiences explained this: for instance, at one time in the concentration camp, the Nazi guards had devised a new game in which they placed before the famished children a glass of milk on the window-ledge, and behind the window there was a machine-gun which they fired. So much the better for the child who, in spite of the machine-gun, managed to get the milk; but two or three died in the attempt.

Peace-time experience of children's groups is not dissimilar. Many modern schools have established a system of self-government among the pre-adolescents, but to do so in a boarding school could be dangerous, if no adults are included in the administration of self-government. It might not be an exaggeration to expect children to be sentenced to death by their comrades, and certainly the severity of the justice of children towards each other will go far beyond the limits of adults' conceptions. Theirs is a justice of violent retribution; of the revenge of the community on the individual.

These pre-adolescents in their concentration camp life were consistent with the general psychological make-up of the 2- and 3-year-olds, and with our knowledge of the unconscious mind of the adult as it reveals itself in dreams, that the only real punishment is capital punishment. If a little child does not like somebody, he wishes that they were dead, that is, out of his life.

Miss Sophie Dann (*who was visiting the Seminar*) spoke of the war-time experiences which Miss Freud had already quoted. The six orphans, who were between 3 and 4 years old, had not wanted to adapt to the new situation at all. They only recognized their own group and they wanted only to live in that group, though a house and everything had been made ready for them by the grown-ups who had thought that the children would be happy to get into new and not hostile surroundings; the children did not want the toys, the food, or the grown-ups. An adult going through the nursery of those six little children might well feel she was not a person, but only air. The important thing to these children was the group, and the grown-ups were there merely to feed and tend the children; it took months to get the children to start to include those few adults into the group. One curious example of the process of inclusion was an occasion when they all bought sweets in a shop and were eating them; then the adult asked that she should be given a sweet, too. They offered the sweets which they had in their mouths and she replied that she would have one when they returned home. Although it was an hour later when they got home, one of them immediately rushed to the sweet box and offered her a substitute sweet.

The recurrence of panic in a group of such children was an interesting phenomenon. They would be getting along quite well and then some disaster, such as one of the children being taken away to hospital, or encountering a dog, would plunge them into panic again. When they first came, they were all afraid of dogs, because one of the watchmen in the German concentration camp used to frighten them with his dog, but gradually they had been persuaded to play with two very small dogs, and they apparently lost their fear within about three months.

About five months later, they were going for a walk on a very lonely path when suddenly an enormous dog came out and stood in front of them. They were exceedingly frightened and screamed. The dog stayed there and one of the children went very white, bit his lip in fear and thought the dog had bitten him. The group was in such a state that it was difficult either to get them on, or to get rid of the dog. After several hours one boy was still quite ill and insisted that the dog had bitten him.

Another instance occurred in this little Sussex village; among the new interests of the children, vehicles were of great importance. One day there came round the corner a big van, used to transport horses, and one little girl got into a dreadful state; she screamed, trembled, and rushed up to it shouting 'Go away, nasty van, awful van!' This must have been a memory from the camp, where people were taken away to the gas chambers in big vans.

Miss Freud added that one of these children, who had gone to America, had retained his fear of dogs, but in his latest photograph he had an enormous dog sitting next to him. While they lived together, group infection accounted for so much that it was difficult to distinguish individual anxiety from shared anxiety.

To return to the subject of adoption: a great deal was done in war-time to match the evacuation home with the social level of the home from which the child had come, and also in adoptions. The evidence of heredity is obscure; and emotionally such matching has not much meaning, because the child's fantasies can convert any kind of home into an ideal home and the best of foster homes into a place of injustice and brutality, or the other way round. The emotional state of the child is of very much greater importance than the actual social conditions.

It is of greater importance to the attitude of the adoptive parents to have a child from their own environment; and, moreover, the demands on a child of a middle-class home of high intellectual level may be very different from those of a working-class home. According to their first upbringing, children are differently prepared to meet such demands. Adoption or placement under good conditions is not always sufficient to put an end to the disturbance of orphans. Is it possible to apply psychoanalysis under such conditions? For therapy to be successful, the child must need it and the adoptive parents wish it. Often adoptive parents do not like interference with their handling of the child; they may have waited a long time for a baby, and they want to try out their own ideas and not share the child with the therapist. The question of therapy in such cases can sometimes be approached in another way: adoption societies, as well as selecting children and safeguarding their conditions, should include among their tasks the psychological preparation of the parents. Begun in the right way, the parents might be grateful enough to the Society to keep in touch with the psychological adviser, whereas they would not make contact with a strange and new clinic.

What should be told to the child, later, about its real mother? A Church Adoption Society in the U.S.A. has the unmarried mother to live with the child for six weeks and nurse her own child; but the more general attitude is that the mother had not exercised her duty of finding the child a father, so the best she could do for it is to give the child up. In this particular agency they have two identical little gold crosses, one of which goes to the mother and one with the baby, to the adoptive parents. When, later on, the child asks the adoptive parents: 'What happened to my mother? Why am I adopted?', the child could be given the replica of the cross which the mother had kept and could be told that its own mother had loved it but could not keep it and so she had sent it with a blessing. This is a symbolic attempt to deal with a very complicated problem; perhaps not an ideal solution, but it indicates the complexities which must be faced in preparing the adoptive parents to answer honestly the questions of the children.

In the United States it is almost universally felt that the child should always be told that it was adopted, and that if the adoptive parents could be equipped with the statement: 'We chose you; other children might just come to their parents but we went and got one; and we wanted a little boy (or girl) and we chose you particularly,' they might then have a way of dealing with inevitable questions.

So far no measure has been found to solve this problem finally. The practice in the U.S.A. has been tried in Britain too, and this explanation may work quite well up to a certain age. If given to the child very early and repeated very often, it might work until the age of 6 or 7. At this age many children form the idea that their real parents are different from their parents with whom they live—that they were born to others, usually, but not always, high-born ones, and that their present parents merely took them over. It might be expected that the adopted child would now come into its own and would feel as the other children, but, on the contrary, the adopted child goes through its greatest upheavals at this age.

With the normal child, these two sets of parents are merely expressions of the child's attitude to his parents at two different ages. The wonderful parents of the fantasy, the fairy story prince and princess, who had given their child to a humble couple to bring up, are merely the parents of the child's own dim past, parents who had seemed so wonderful then. The child carries in its mind two images of his parents: the image appropriate to the infant, of the all-powerful parent; and then the diminished image appropriate to the child going to school, whose parents have begun to take on the natural dimensions of human beings, with their faults and possibilities of error.

Just as the normal child's longings, at 6 or 7 years, go back to those imaginary parents of the past, so the interest of the adopted child goes away from the adoptive parents to the real ones who have deserted him, but instead of finding wonderful parents, the adopted child can only find a mother who had given him up. It can be an enormous shock to the child, to find no wonderful image of the mother. The danger at that time may be that adopted children will actually look for their real parents. For instance, a little boy from Miss Dann's home, who had been adopted in America, now wanted to return to England and look for his real parents because he had been told that they were lost in the war. Other children wander about in search of their lost parents, and the image of the lost parents has great power in their lives. So far, short of approaching it in therapy, no means has emerged of altering that situation and it is not certain how far it can be done by therapy.

The question of phantom parents may be important among children conceived by artificial insemination; is the parental attitude communicable to the child? It is difficult to determine the extent to which children react to the unexpressed attitudes of their parents. The child adopted because of the father's infertility (and in many cases the child produced by artificial insemination) will always mean to the father, apart from his loving and wanting the child, a living sign of his impotence or sterility, of which no man likes to be reminded. This, surely, must impart itself to the child in some manner or degree.

A peculiarly unfortunate, though not uncommon, situation arises when the mother of a child recently adopted, becomes pregnant. Why that should happen is a matter for psychological, obstetrical and endocrinological speculation, but it is a fairly well-known fact that some mothers conceive after years of sterility, within a few months of adopting a baby. In that situation the parent had the living sign of impotence or sterility there, for nothing as it were. Such a situation can be potentially dangerous to the whole family.

There used to be a law in Austria that adoption was not permitted to a woman who could still produce a child; quite in contrast to the practice in many other countries, where the mother must be of child-bearing age. The latter is certainly the case in the United Kingdom, but in the Netherlands adoption is illegal and cannot be undertaken, and in the Irish Republic adoption was made legal only in 1952.

Dr. Soddy, in concluding the discussion, said that some psychiatrists were feeling their way towards a concept of psychosis in young children, in terms of a gross failure to connect with the world, as it were, at various ages and various levels. Could one regard feeding and sleeping difficulties, particularly in children before weaning, as possible evidence of a lack of orientation, particularly of orientation in time? Out of this lack of orientation to the rhythms of life something very fundamental in the genesis of a psychosis may appear. There are also curious phenomena of neurological development which appear to become disjointed and to lose the rhythm of life, without necessarily any particular effect on intelligence. The whole picture builds up into the kind of child some call deviant or abnormal, in whose aetiology separation and other early disasters are commonplace.

Miss Freud, summing up, drew attention to the many untapped sources of information which exist in all countries. The practice of collecting children in institutions may cease within a measurable period of years, for it has already been reduced to a great extent, to the great advantage of the children; but institutions, orphanages, foundling homes, and so on, still survive, and the opportunity should be taken of studying institutional life and the ego development of the children in those institutions. Wherever children live in their own natural families, no stranger can really enter their life and study them, whereas children are open to study in an institution. As the material might cease to exist, we must not omit to use it while it is still available.

One further point: it is now known that the visual and the acoustic impressions which a child receives in the first years of life from his close contact with the mother, and those of the following years received from the father and other members of the family, contribute the major part of what later becomes his personality. This is a reason for studying the personality development in children with visual and auditory defects. In this way the relative importance of the various sense impressions can be determined.

160

Part Four

DIFFERENT CULTURAL PATTERNS AND TECHNOLOGICAL CHANGE

FAMILY AND CHILD DEVELOPMENT
PATTERNS
IN OTHER CULTURES

Margaret Mead

HOWEVER FAR BACK we go in human history, we always find the family. There is no human society in the world without it and no human society has succeeded in abolishing it permanently.

However, some very strange things have been done with the family in a little island called Mentawei, off the coast of Sumatra. There, the head of the family is so important that he is virtually a priest and cannot work. He cannot marry, therefore, until he has a son old enough to do the work. This dilemma is met by keeping all relationships secret. As children are born they are adopted by their maternal grandmother, and the young maternal uncles do all the work and support the children. Then, as soon as a son becomes old enough to do the work, the father marries the mother, adopts his children, and sets up housekeeping—rather late but nevertheless respectable.

Among the Nairs of Malabar, the men very much object to having the women under the dominance of a man outside the family, so the children are all married very young and divorced the same day. The women live at home with their parents and have lovers who have no social standing in the family; the men keep full control over their sisters and their sisters' children.

These are peculiar, extreme cases, but from the study of extreme cases in social organization we learn the limits to which human society can go. There are still societies in which the men look after the children and protect them, although comparative studies of the anthropoid apes lead us to believe that there is no inborn instinct of fatherhood. It is the task of society to invent ways of making men willing to be fathers, in the social sense. Society has to devise ways of persuading its young men that it is a good and desirable thing to marry, have children, and spend their lives looking after them.

Among the Mundugumor of New Guinea a man can have several wives if he is strong enough. A very strong man can get many wives. In another tribe, the Arapesh, although monogamy is the rule, many men have two wives because they have to care for the wives

163

of their older brothers or cousins who have died. Each wife is treated as if she were the only one, has a house of her own, and thinks her husband should spend all his time with her. So it is possible for a community to have an ideal for the family which few people can attain, while all the others act as if they had that kind of family.

Periodically in history, these devices break down and the family goes to pieces: then the mother-child unit is scattered about, supported by the state, by other relatives, or by the mother alone. However, no society lasts for long if the family is completely broken up, even in the case of minority groups. Among the Negro Americans in the United States, whose family life during slave days was completely destroyed, there were temporary marriages, but the master might sell the wife, the husband, and the children, all in different directions. The mothers and mothers' mothers would look after the children, and the men came and went. It was not until Negroes became citizens that the Negro family reconstituted itself. It is a common occurrence among workers who have emigrated to a more advanced country for the family to break up for a time, but later to recover. There is no record whatever of any society surviving without the family unit within it.

The Nazi experiment was an experiment against the family; the regime gave strong support to the unmarried mother. During the early days of the Soviet Union there was an attempt to get rid of the family, but the striking sequel has been the reconstitution of the family. The Soviet Union has to-day one of the most puritanical family set-ups in the Western world, with the least tolerance for divorce and the strongest demands on parents. Women are expected to work and bring up their children at the same time.

In studying any family system one should ask how adequately it is bringing up the next generation to rear families. The family has to prepare boys to be willing to be husbands and fathers, and girls to be willing to be wives and mothers. Many societies, both in Asia and in the West, have survived with a large monastic group, but a certain bulk of the population has to be willing to be responsible for carrying on the race. There has been a tendency to think of the family as being based on sex activity, but the exclusive possession of a female by a male is found even among the great apes. The strongest males have the females they want, and other males have what they can get. That which distinguishes humanity is that the father provides the food, for among the great apes he does not feed the pregnant or lactating female or his children. Among the great apes the male progenitor has a sexual and protective role, not a nutritive role.

With the innovation of food-getting for the family by the males, the family can be said to have begun. Perhaps that is the reason why people defend the family meal so vigorously, why family meals are felt to be so sacred. The gathering of the family for the family meal, to consume the food which the father has provided, and the mother has prepared, can be regarded as very basic in the history of the family.

In the West, a fear is sometimes expressed that the family will disappear, while in some of the Near Eastern countries there is a fear that the family is too strong. It is important to realize that the family is very tough. It is the strongest institution in society, but it needs to change in relation to the changes which are going on in society.

To-day it seems to us that the family composed of a mother-child unit, without a father, is pathological and subhuman, no matter how many medical services or social schemes support it. To turn the role of the father into that of a paying agency and deputize his role to nurses, health visitors, midwives, paediatricians and obstetricians, is a form of pathology in society which has occurred in different ways in the past but against which society will probably rebel. At least, that is what the anthropologist concludes at present.

The family not only protects and feeds the child while it is young and dependent, but it teaches the child its male or female role. Within the family situation, a girl can learn to become a woman and a boy to become a man.

The Chinese people think that every little baby needs some person to look after it all the time, perhaps an elder sister or a grandmother, and under such a system, the mother or the nurse learns to understand the baby very well. They watch the baby's face and toilet-train the child by learning the rhythms of its expressions, the way its muscles move. This practice is neither conditioned-reflex training, nor is the child left until it is old enough to understand. It is entirely dependent upon having a grown-up person or an elder child to spend all her time attending to the little child. Such a system would not be possible in a modern American or English family with a mother and even two small children, with all her own work to do.

One of the difficulties of the family in the modern world is the change in its form from the rural family to the urban family, or from the European family to the American family. In a time of reorientation, people may be brought up in the kind of family in which they will not continue to live as adults. It can be hard for a girl who grew up in a comfortable family group with a grandmother, aunts and cousins coming in and out, where there was always somebody to talk to, to move to a little flat or a house on a housing estate.

She has no technique for holding one baby under one arm and the other baby under the other while answering the telephone! She comes from a society where there have been other people to do things for her.

One of the reasons why we have to have so many books on child-care and mothercraft to-day, and Mental Health Congresses, is because people have grown up in one kind of family and have to live in another. Only too often, also, the husband grew up in one kind of family and the wife in another. Either he does not want her to be like his mother and she does not want him to be like her father, or else they do, and in either case they are both likely to be disappointed.

Some may think that I over-emphasize the role of social environment as compared with that of heredity; that there is an organic type of person who would make a polygamist and another constitutional type who would make a monogamist; or even a third type, more rare, which would be well-suited to polyandry, that is, several husbands with one wife. But people of the same stock and ancestry are able to change their form of family; on one side of the mountain one may find polygamy and on the other monogamy, and they can be interchanged.

It is known that people of the same stock and ancestry can live in a great many different family forms, and there are instances of families which, in three generations, have moved from the family form of nomad tribes in Asia to the flat-dwelling, telephone-answering family of England and America, without any alteration in physical type. Such families produce extraordinarily different types of character in succeeding generations; all the difference between that of a child who has only his father and mother and perhaps one sibling at home, and that of a child brought up in a family of twenty or thirty people.

Orphan children who have grown up in an institution are able to marry later, because they learn from other people about fathers and mothers and families, and come to want a family of their own. Sometimes children reared in institutions make very good marriages because they partake in the pattern favoured in their society.

The same thing is true about brother and sister relationships. The way in which parents handle brother and sister relationships will make an enormous difference in the character of the developing child.

I have made a film[1] of two different ways of handling jealousy, which illustrates how different these things may look in different cultures. By looking at contrasting ways of doing things, one can

[1] *Childhood Rivalry in Bali and New Guinea.* See Film List, p. 297.

get a good deal more insight into one's own customs, while the advantage of using primitive material for illustration is its greater distance from all of us.

Dr. Mead then showed the film Childhood Rivalry.

The film showed Karba's mother handling another baby and inciting the child's jealousy, and other Balinese mothers' attempts to mute the jealousy where the child's own sibling was concerned. The Balinese do not tolerate unkindness to brothers and sisters. When Karba was given a doll he rejected it.

The second part of the film showed scenes in New Guinea of another way of meeting jealousy, this time by the mother attending to the older child who was in competition with the baby for food and for everything to do with the mother. The result is strong identification with the mother by both boys and girls, and though the New Guinea boys become head-hunters by very late identification with the father, the rituals of the New Guinea society are concerned with men pretending to be women. In contrast, in Western Europe one hears of little girls wanting to be little boys.

The New Guinea ceremonial is concerned with men pretending to have children, and they have many ceremonies in which they imitate maternal functions. We have no reason to believe that these people differ in physical endowment from any other group of people. In every group there are great differences between individuals—there are stupid ones, bright ones, thin ones, fat ones, people whose temper is quick and people whose temper is slow, children who walk early and children who walk late, children who are verbal and children who are not. The only difference in variation from that found among children in the Western world, is that you do not find mentally defective children, because if they are not killed soon after birth, they die later because of their deficiency and the lack of medical care.

There is no clear reason for assigning differences between cultures to heredity but there is good reason to conclude that different kinds of family patterns, different ways of treating children, develop different patterns of adjustment to the environment. Of any family system we can ask: does it arrange to produce the number of children that that society feels it needs? This is very different from seeking to save the number of children that a society believes should be saved. There are many societies, of course, with both female infanticide and polygamy. Societies give to the children the character which they are expected to have and which they need to prepare them for adult life, marriage and old age—all these later periods of life being prefigured within the family by the way the children are brought up.

167

In the changing world we have to work for the sort of family which is capable of change, so that if the father and mother move from the country to the city or from one country to another, they are able to adjust their relationship so as to survive the change and to bring up children who are able to live in a changing world, able to tolerate the fact that their own children will behave in a way they never saw. What we ask modern parents to do is to bring up an unknown child, the kind of child they have never seen, so that it can live in an unknown world.

DISCUSSION

Although there was a population of a little under one million in Bali, there was no mental hospital on the island (1936–39). The people have a very high tolerance of insane behaviour, provided it is not violent, and of mental deficiency.

Among the Iatmul of New Guinea, there are strong cultural influences in the direction of homosexuality, as may be inferred from the fact that the language includes eleven words for sodomy. On those occasions when small boys make homosexual advances or have homosexual relations, the bigger boys immediately separate them, give them a stick each and make them fight it out instead. The effect of this and of the community attitude is that boys grow up in the belief that homosexuality is desirable; but there are no passive men in the community because every one who shows signs of passivity is given a big stick and is expected to fight. Homosexuality is, therefore, near the surface all the time, but is manifested in aggression rather than in sex.

The appearance of such behaviour as fraternal jealousy can never be ascribed solely to the behaviour of the mother to the child. However much the mother may live a secluded life, her relationship with other human beings is always present, in the tone of her voice and in the whole way in which she tends the child. For this reason it can be said that the cause of adult jealousy lies in the whole society, and in everybody's past.

A curious feature of this New Guinea society is that the children of the less-favoured wife are usually the better adjusted. This may be due to the extent to which the favoured wife would be distracted from her children by the attention of her husband.

Erik Erikson in his book *Childhood and Society* (9) emphasizes the importance of knowing what a child must learn at different ages. Different family systems in different parts of the world meet these problems in different ways. Families which begin training their children to be clean from birth are treating the new-born baby as if it were a 2-year-old. The common American practice of lecturing even the 6-month-old baby and telling him what to do, is more appropriate for a much older age. By contrast, in societies such as the Arapesh of New Guinea a child will often be carried until it is 3 or 4 years old. It is interesting that these people are physically clumsy; they take a passive attitude towards tools, and handle them very badly. In other parts of New Guinea, children will be perfectly agile at 15 months.

A valuable key to a society is to find out the major kinds of sanction, positive and negative, which are used in the family system. Societies like Bali depend on fear for character formation. Some societies use shame and pride as their principle sanction. Pride is the training of the aristocrat who is being brought up to be a gentleman. Others continually invoke the neighbours in some form or another and this, the approval or disapproval of the tribe, is possibly the most powerful sanction of all; it is quite capable of causing death from shame amongst those tribes that use it. It is possible to teach slightly older children that the parents will withdraw their love or punish them if they do something wrong, and this goes on to produce the type of character with internal sanctions, people who will behave themselves whatever the environment is like.

It is important to remember that in most societies there are many variations. Even in Bali, where there is a very uniform picture, there was one mother who deviated from the normal pattern of under-developed secondary sexual characteristics. She had large pendulous breasts, and was a plump, comfortable, warm woman. Her children were exceedingly plump and comfortable, too. It was found that her children were, according to the Gesell norms, the two most physically advanced children in the community.

The main contribution of anthropology to these studies is to give a sense of how things are inter-related and to show the importance of small details in comparing different societies. In this way changes can be made carefully and responsibly, with the realization that changes in one area of a person's life will probably mean changes in other areas.

Anthropology also gives some idea of the untapped potentialities of human beings. It may show the things human beings are capable of doing which they do not realize they can do.

CULTURAL DIFFERENCES IN THE BATHING OF BABIES

Margaret Mead

AT THE FIRST SESSION of the Seminar, as an introduction to the method of teaching, and an exercise in the observation of human behaviour, Dr. Margaret Mead showed a film entitled *Bathing Babies in three Cultures*[1]. She explained that the word 'culture' was used in this title in the technical sense given to it by American and English anthropologists, with the meaning of the total behaviour of any group of people, and that the 'cultural pattern' of a people includes such common activities as the manner in which they bake their bread, get married or bury their dead. Observers of unfamiliar scenes can make many mistakes in attempting to analyse their data unless they are in possession of all the facts and can recognize the 'pattern' or design inherent in the whole situation.

In the film, scenes from three types of culture are shown. The first, a primitive tribe of New Guinea, the Iatmul, until recently head-hunters; the second, an expensive suburb in Hollywood; and the third, the island of Bali in the Dutch East Indies, where the culture is similar in some respects to that of Europe in the Middle Ages. Babies of the same age in each of these settings were taken as the subject of the demonstration.

In the New Guinea scene, the mother, firmly grasping the child by the arm, plunges it from a steep bank into a river infested with crocodiles; the Hollywood mother baths her baby in a well-equipped bathroom and the baby's attention is distracted with toys; while the Balinese woman is seen gently washing her child in a tub. Dr. Mead pointed out how the American child's attention is directed away from his personal relationship to his mother by the toys. In the New Guinea society, the parents encourage the child towards a strong, independent, assertive sort of life; and both in New Guinea and in Bali the child is fed when it is hungry and for as long as it is hungry. The New Guinea mother insists on the child showing how hungry it is before she feeds it. It has to show that it has energy enough to demand food.

The mothers of the New Guinea and Bali children do not talk to their children as much as, for example, an English or an Eastern

[1] See Film List, p. 297.

170

European Jewish mother might talk to hers. The greater expressiveness of the hands in the shots taken in New Guinea and Bali, as compared with those of the American mother, are also interesting. The average American woman may never hold a little baby until she nurses her own, and even then she often behaves as though she were still afraid that the infant might break in her hands. In New Guinea and Bali, on the contrary, they know all about babies. Small infants are looked after by child nurses as young as 4 years old, and this familiarity is shown in all their movements.

There are other differences among mothers, for example, in the degree to which they insist on good behaviour in the baby. The English mother may simply put her hand out without speaking, in the endeavour to prevent the baby from doing something she does not want it to do, whereas the American mother would give it a long lecture. In Bali also, as soon as the baby is born, a pattern of behaviour to which it is supposed to adhere, is imposed upon it. As far as we know the chronological stages of development of the child are the same everywhere, and the children of the simplest and most complicated people alike, start out with the same potentialities and the same possibilities of learning.

One of the difficulties in mental hygiene all over the world is that the idealists tend to ignore the existence of cultural patterns. For example, the peasant woman newly arrived in the United States will smack her baby when it annoys her, and feed it when it cries. Then the public-health nurse will come and teach her not to feed it when it cries, but according to a time-schedule. She does not, however, make any change in the practice of smacking the baby, and thus the whole pattern is thrown out of balance. Similarly, believing that it is good to feed babies on a schedule, people try to introduce schedule-feeding everywhere—in Burma and Tibet, as well as in London and New York. They try, in fact, to make universal something which may be good in one place but not good in another, and to take the practice of highly civilized communities as a universal rule, regardless of the way in which it may upset the balance of the local cultural pattern.

BIRTH OF A BABY IN NEW GUINEA

Margaret Mead

INTRODUCING A FILM on the birth of a baby in New Guinea,[1] Dr. Margaret Mead said that it had been taken during 1938 in the tribe shown in one of the episodes in the film of the babies being bathed.

The film shows the treatment of an infant from a moment before the cord was cut and just after the birth. The mother had started to run to the village to fetch tobacco for her husband, and the child was born suddenly, in a little wood behind the village.

The film illustrates a mother-child relationship unencumbered by clothes. The infant wears nothing, and the mother wears only two little grass aprons, one in front and one behind. The extent to which the infant is ready to suck right after the birth can be seen. In this tribe a wet-nurse, usually a woman nursing a baby less than six months old, is brought to suckle the child for the first twenty-four hours or so, until the mother has milk. After about twenty-four hours the baby is given to the mother, but if she does not have enough milk the suckling by the wet-nurse continues.

The influence of early feeding on later thumb-sucking is of interest, for nowhere, as far as is known, is there thumb-sucking among primitive people not influenced by Western behaviour. Finger sucking may occur later, but not thumb-sucking. Dr. Mead had seen one infant only who started to suck his thumb, and that was in New Guinea on an occasion when there was no wet-nurse available for several hours. In those hours that infant had found his thumb, but he did not continue to suck it. There is a possibility that thumb-sucking, as compared with finger-sucking, is established very early.

The cord was cut with a piece of bamboo and tied with a little piece of strong grass, similar to the raffia used for weaving. If the baby had been born in the bush, the mother would have taken a little piece off her grass skirt to tie it.

The fact that the mother apparently very carefully wiped off the natural protective covering of the baby and then replaced it with mud reinforces the suggestion that there is no instinctive behaviour left among human beings. There are cases where either the mother or the father bites the cord in two, which must naturally always be done if there is no knife, bamboo, or nutshell; but to do so is also

[1] *First Days in the Life of a New Guinea Baby*. See Film List, p. 297.

172

highly artificial behaviour, old in history, although it may look instinctive. This mother wiped off all of the original fluid and then twenty minutes later put on some clay—exactly the same technique as used in Western cultures.

The placenta was placed in a coco-nut shell which was buried at the foot of a coco-nut tree. In almost every society the placenta is treated very carefully, and often something is done to determine the child's future industry, according to the sex. A girl's placenta may be put near a weaving tool or a pestle and mortar, while a boy's would be put near a hunting weapon or a tool.

The practice of suckling shortly after birth varies from tribe to tribe. In Samoa, where on the whole very good relations exist between parent and child, they will not let the baby nurse until they are sure there is real milk; there is no wet-nurse. On the other hand in Bali there is a wet-nurse at once; and there are many places where the infant is put directly to the mother's breast at birth, and it simply sucks until finally it gets some milk.

Practice regarding midwives also varies. In many cultures there are two or three old women in the village who are better midwives than the others and to whom most people would go, but in one of the New Guinea tribes the midwife is always the woman who has most recently had a baby.

LIFE IN BALI

Margaret Mead

THE CARE of the baby has been very much emphasized at the Seminar, but many people may feel that, after all, babies have grown up during the last hundred thousand years in spite of the most extraordinary conditions. For example, among the nomadic Lapps the baby born at night has a better chance of survival than the baby born by day, when the people are on the move, and there is no chance of rest for the mother.

Physical conditions vary greatly but psychological conditions vary even more. Children may be brought up under conditions which most psychiatrists would think shockingly bad. In some cultures it is thought to be good upbringing for a baby to be treated badly, otherwise it would not know how to behave when it grows up. Study of punishments has shown that people tend to use as punishment those deprivations from which they themselves suffered in childhood, but it is not only in the field of deprivation and punishment that the life of an infant is related to the life of the adult in the same society.

The exposure of an infant to a situation which fills it with rage and guilt can be a preparation for what is expected to come later. The development in an infant of a desire to hit its father or mother can be an appropriate preparation for a religion which uses sin as a way of communicating with God. There are religions which say that the man who has never sinned does not know about God. In all societies with their own religious, artistic, and philosophical systems, the treatment meted out to the child is related to, and is a preparation for, adulthood.

Adults, as they handle children, carry within themselves the impulses to appropriate behaviour. The American baby who is not picked up when it cries will later hear the preacher in church emphasize the value of self-control and so-called 'good' behaviour as a means to salvation. The mother, as she lets the baby cry, will believe that she is helping it towards these virtues and this reward.

The emphasis laid in recent times on what happens in the first two years is closely related to the fact that we can no longer predict what will happen to the child when it grows up. Living in a changing world, nobody knows whether the child will be able to follow the

174

religion of its parents; whether, for example, if it is prepared for the kind of religion where sin is relieved by confession, it will become a member of a Church which will permit it to confess. Children are launched on an unknown sea, and by giving the small infant the best possible start, we hope to prepare it for whatever it may have to face later on.

At the same time, of course, every society has political, religious, and artistic institutions which serve to meet the needs developed in childhood. For sibling-rivalry, in Anglo-Saxon countries they provide football, cricket, or baseball matches, in which it is possible for the players to be as aggressive as they would like to be with their brothers and sisters, and a large part of the population obtains from organized sports, as players or spectators, the satisfaction it needs. Wherever we turn we find some such correspondence as the correspondence in Japan between the position of the Emperor and that of the father, though somebody has said that since the Emperor of Japan's position was altered the status of all the fathers in Japan has deteriorated, because the father was the representative of the Emperor in the family. In Anglo-Saxon countries there is certainly a correspondence between two parents in the home and two-party systems of government, and perhaps one of the requisites of two-party systems is a reasonably strong mother; whereas one-party systems are symbolical of the idea of the supreme overriding authority of the father.

The films of Bali[1] are sufficiently remote to permit of a good degree of detachment in viewing. They show the way in which a Balinese child is reared, from the age of 6 months to 2 years, and those who are experienced in the effect of parental behaviour on young children will be quite surprised but will be able to make predictions as to what should happen to a child treated like this. It should be realized that this is the way that all Balinese children are treated.

The father and mother shown in the films approximate closely to the Balinese ideal of men and women. The ideal Balinese woman is cold, slim, and distant; the ideal Balinese man is a little more like a puppy, a little warmer and woollier than the woman. The Balinese are among the most contented people in the world. Visitors from America and Europe go away describing a sort of paradise. They talk of people who hardly know what fatigue is, who run rather than walk, who have a good co-operative system of irrigation, so that the average Balinese has almost three times as much to eat as the average Javanese. They have practically eliminated war; every individual participates in the arts; there is not a minute of the day

---

[1] *Karba's First Years* and *Dance and Trance in Bali*. See Film List, p. 297.

or night when the air is not filled with music. Even at midnight a lonely performer will be heard playing his musical instrument. The pigeons have bells attached to their feet so that as they wheel over the village they make music. The housewife works with a knife with little bells on the end which jingle.

Every detail of daily life is accompanied by offerings. They never cook a meal without making little offerings. Food is prepared for the gods and eaten by the mortals. They make beautiful cakes, take them to the temple, leave a bit of essence and then take the cake home to eat. If they have been lucky in the markets or at gambling they give a theatrical performance as an offering to the gods, which all the people of the village enjoy. It is an extraordinarily well-integrated, very peaceful, very artistic society. The people spend hours in the fields by day, and half the night rehearsing for a theatrical show.

Ceremonials occur again and again which make meaningful the kind of experience which the child has had. Some societies arouse in children no needs that cannot easily be met; some develop in the children a complex of needs which can nevertheless be fulfilled; and others develop in children a variety of desires which there is no way to meet.

The first film, *Karba's First Years*, opened with a birthday ceremony when the baby had his hair cut for the first time, at 6 months old. At $10\frac{1}{2}$ months he has his first lesson in walking, and at 1 year he has his first music lesson on an instrument like a xylophone. At 13 months he is seen holding on to a single rail; at 14 months balancing himself in his tub. The Balinese children learn both to dance and to play musical instruments before they can walk.

There are several scenes showing the parents teasing the child, at which he goes into a temper and screams. The recurrent experience of a Balinese child is that of broken climax; the mother starts to play with or caress him and then loses interest and turns away. As the child gets a little older, his parents' play gets much harsher. His mother tries to make him jealous, so when he starts to play with other children he is sulky and unresponsive. Later he will grow up to be gay like all Balinese but never again responsive to another person's behaviour.

The second film, *Dance and Trance in Bali*, showed a conflict between a witch and a dragon, an often-recurring theme that every Balinese child sees many times during its life. The witch treats the other dancers just as the mother does the child. She is unresponsive and turns her back on them, but when they attack her they are not strong enough to overcome her. The dragon represents the friendlier and warmer father.

176

The Balinese child is treated by its parents in a way that most psychiatrists would think very bad, but the child sees, on the stage, the attack on the witch, the attack that the child never made on its mother, and sees that the witch does not die. The dragon is the protector of life, and the witch represents death and fear.

Emotions not permitted in real life are continuously enacted on the Balinese stage. This is not a matter of someone having an unhappy childhood and growing up to write a novel about it, but the continuous contemporary re-enactment of every child's unhappiness and frustration.

On a test devised for schizophrenics in the West, the Balinese yielded results indistinguishable from the schizophrenics'. But these Balinese get married, become parents of children, and live a completely integrated life in their own community. Balinese society can support a large amount of schizophrenic behaviour without recourse to segregation.

When the Balinese are frustrated or frightened they go to sleep. If the village council meets to decide whether to turn a thief over to the Government, the accused may go to sleep while the old men debate. If the house-servants forget something very important they all go to sleep. They meet every real situation by withdrawal, but they have available to them in their religion and ceremonial a continuous stream of ways in which they can act out, in group ceremonial, the fears and frustrations of childhood.

Because of the way in which the culture of Bali is organized, the children are secure. In changing societies one can probably never invent daily ceremonials to fit so perfectly the frustrations of childhood; and in lieu of such inventions all that can be done is to try to avoid for the children a crippling series of frustrations which will require, in turn, the most elaborate and special kinds of adult political and religious life.

DISCUSSION

Delinquency is not a serious problem in Bali. Society is organized so tightly that the little municipalities enforce their own laws, and if these are not adhered to, the persons concerned become vagrant. Vagrancy, and consequently theft, are the most usual forms of crime, and violence is extremely rare.

There is a great deal of laxity concerning belief in religion, which has been described as a religion which nobody believes in but which everybody enjoys. On the whole people are more concerned about breaking the rules of their own village than of any general rules of religion. The principal sins punished in this society are incest and marrying into the wrong caste. It is possible to expiate sins in the

N   177

next world, and because of the system of reincarnation nothing is final or permanently terrifying, although there is a good deal in the culture which is frightening in a recurrent way.

There is a very similar ritual dance in Algeria among a sect called 'tremblers'. The dance, as usually performed, is largely composed of a trance in which a number of dangerous things are done, such as walking over red-hot coals, and it goes on until the dancers fall to the ground exhausted. Meanwhile their leader, who is a sheik with a good deal of religious authority, presides over the occasion in a serene and reassuring way, and revives the dancers when they fall into a trance by making them breathe a powder of incense and tobacco and by reciting incantations. This dance appeared to meet the same deep need as the trance and dance in Bali, by giving the onlookers an image of control of the wild elements in evil and death, by a good figure of serenity and power.

There is a great deal in common between the behaviour of these people in the dance with that of hypnotic subjects, and in particular the look of strain and agony on the faces of the subjects during the trance is typical. Also, people in this sort of trance undoubtedly can do painful and intricate things to themselves and to each other, but the striking feature of this trance behaviour is that it is always strictly controlled. People are not allowed to be violent and even the behaviour which looks the most uncontrolled is, in fact, done by the right man at the right place in the dance.

The arousal of jealousy in their sons by Bali mothers resembles a series of games rather than a routine of character formation. For example, a child might perhaps be threatened that the mother would die or that he would be given to another mother. Everybody plays these games and they have no idea why they do it.

Not enough is known about Balinese history really to understand the origin of all these practices. The dragon comes from China, and the witch from Hinduism. There are also Mohammedan influences at a later date. Their history does not explain the development of this particular type of behaviour. Their prosperity and lack of hunger leaves them with time to go in for elaborate ceremonial. By contrast, the Australian aboriginal has to spend so much of his time seeking food that this type of behaviour does not exist. The Balinese have, in fact, solved the problem of leisure, which bears so heavily upon a Western community now that there is an eight-hour working day.

There are no detailed records of other societies bringing up their children in this fashion, though many societies have evil figures. In France, for example, there is a frightening man who will take bad children away in a bag. There is no parallel frightening female figure in the French system. Another interesting difference is that although the European attitude towards God is that of a child towards its father, the Balinese, on the other hand, call their gods children. In Bali, the word for serving the god, serving the king, or spoiling the baby, is the same, and there is a relationship between servant and master, people and gods, parents and babies, which is almost the reverse of the European relationship.

It is surprising how, in view of the fact that the children are teased, left unpacified, and encouraged to react with rage, there is so little neurotic behaviour among adults, but there is a good deal of disassociation and aloofness. Another interesting result is the lack of climax in their lives and in their art. A Balinese love affair is much like a meeting between total strangers in which the man would think of the woman not as his mother, but as a beautiful fair princess. The real climax in the affair is the first interchange of looks. Consummation is not felt to be as exciting as the first moment, and in fact, strong pressures have to be used in this society to make people marry. There is an unduly high proportion of old bachelors and even of old maids. An ideal arrangement is to have a house in the village and another on the farm, with husband and wife living separately. They tend to avoid responsibilities in marriage and there are recurrent extra-marital relationships with strangers. It is typical that in the theatre the wife, the mother-in-law and the ugly princess are dressed exactly alike, and whereas the man hopes to marry the princess, he makes a mistake and usually gets the ugly duckling, as it were, who is dressed just like his mother.

THE EFFECTS OF TECHNOLOGICAL CHANGE ON CHILD DEVELOPMENT

Margaret Mead

MANY OF THE PEOPLE who are interested in this subject are concerned with newly industrialized countries, and some would like to study definite techniques which could be used in the introduction of change in their own societies. They will find useful a manual called *Cultural Patterns and Technical Change* (18) published by UNESCO in French and English, though some of the details in it may already be out of date, since there were considerable delays in publication. I want, in this paper, to discuss a general way of looking at technological change and its implications for mental health and child development.

About fifty years ago, sociologists (20) decided that all technological change was of a different order from other kinds of change. They decided that it must be cumulative, because they believed that invention in the fields of mechanics, transportation, agriculture and use of power, proceeded cumulatively. According to this theory, technological change could be recorded by a line rising very steeply, whereas in the fields of human relations, family life, or forms of educational and religious institutions, change occurred by abandoning one form in favour of another. In the thinking of this period, technology might go from water power to steam power to electric power and, finally, to atomic power, but the family remained, on the whole, static. Polygamy could change to monogamy, and vice versa, but they could not exist together. In this field nothing was cumulative, there was only simple alternation and substitution.

This view seemed exceedingly plausible twenty-five years ago. The students of that period regarded matters such as public health, social work, or psychiatry as what they termed 'adaptive culture', a social invention to cope with the difference between the high rate of change in man's control of the natural world and his slow rate of change in other respects. This gave rise to a vision of a world which was going to get more and more unmanageable and which would need more and more social workers to patch up differences, as the rate of technological change became faster and faster.

180

However, a great deal of the original interest in social anthropology came from making these observations. We now talk about the relationship of the public health movement to industrialization in Britain, about how the young mother, separated from her background and parents, was handicapped in home and child care, and how the public health service stepped in to fill the gap; whereas fifty years ago we should have talked about the slum mothers and would have believed that the slums were filled with depravity. Focusing attention on inventions has made enormous contributions to our awareness of social processes, to our knowledge of the dependence of the mother on the grandmother and the difficulty of replacing that tie, and to our knowledge of how dependent even married women once were. We could see that a certain method of bringing up children worked very nicely so long as the bringing up of adolescents and the forms of marriage fitted together. But when change became so rapid that children were reared in one way, went to school in another, went to work in another, and got married in still another way, human beings could not be depended on to function as they had in the past.

It is interesting to note that while the United Nations refer to under-developed countries, no one talks about over-developed countries. There seems to be an assumption that every country in the world is under- or over- something, instead of working at different rates of change, though more and more in relation to each other. It is striking that some of the so-called economically under-developed countries are among the oldest in civilization and have conserved many things which the over-developed countries have never had. The words 'under-' or 'over-developed' 'mature' or 'immature', are not very satisfactory. The word 'industrialization' can be used to refer to a country which has a lot of factories in which people work for wages, in contrast to a national economy based on agriculture and village industries. The countries most recently industrialized can still gain a great deal by studying the effects of rapid change, by discussing what happens to the people who move from the country to the city, what happens when they crowd together without sanitation, after being accustomed to the country way of life where the children, the chickens, the lambs, all got on happily together. It is commonly said that the habitual way of life becomes altered in the cities in ways that we do not recognize, that it means a loss of religion, a loss of what we are pleased to call superstition—that is, the things other people believe in and we do not—but it may be doubted whether the average English or American attitude to a vitamin is very different from the average savage's attitude to a good or evil spirit.

It would pay those who are working in newly industrialized

countries or recently rural areas to keep in mind how dramatic are the changes accompanying technological change, which accompany the shift from human power to machine power. At the same time it is important to realize that the social analysts of fifty years ago said that there were two kinds of change: a cumulative kind concerned with man's natural environment, and a non-cumulative or substantive kind concerned with man's relations to himself, to his fellows, and to the universe. That assumption failed to take account of the fact that each human being carries his culture within himself. Man went into the factory, where he had to work differently, attuned to the clock instead of to the rhythm of his own heart, but he was the same man.

A man living in a changing society becomes himself a creature of change. Though human beings change if they have been reared in one situation and then have to work in another, character remains. The people who have learned to live in change and those who have not, continue to illustrate the theories of fifty years ago in that they have had to make a different kind of liaison with their environment. Most of our inventions such as social work, public health, education for mothercraft, are the outcome of the period when people continued to assume that they came from one place which was fixed and had to get to another place which was fixed, and in between they read a book or got psychoanalysed to help them get from one place to another—so that they could stand still again. It is this feeling which underlies the nostalgic looking back to the golden days. Older people among us look back to the period before 1914, to life in a nursery where all the furniture had rounded corners, and younger people look back at the world before World War II, but all must cope with the fact that they are living in a different, and to them deteriorated, state of society.

We have learned an enormous amount from the practice of giving a mother a book when her own mother was absent, and we have learned a lot from modern psychiatry, especially from psychoanalysis, but all this learning has come from people suffering from social change. It is doubtful if one could psychoanalyse a perfectly happy member of a static society even if he wanted to be psychoanalysed. To-day we deal continuously with people who bear within them the imprint of disharmony, who are in the midst of social change which their upbringing does not help them to face.

The Bali film[1] illustrates the fact that human society has survived, that parents do peculiar things to their children, but that a society which has a ritual and beliefs that help the children, can survive. If there is a religious system which stresses dependence, the whole

---

[1] *A Balinese Family.* See Film List, p. 297.

society may be dependent; the priest will be a father, and the rituals will accentuate the sense of sin. Quite stable people can be produced out of methods of feeding and toilet-training that seem terrible to us. There may be social devices which compensate for such methods of child-training. It all depends upon the stability of the society, and circumstances are very different when infants are being brought up to live in change.

The recognition that technological change and other changes do not proceed at different rates introduces a different principle: that of recognizing changes other than those resulting from the pressure of technological change upon character. Once the wheel was invented things could be moved which human beings could not carry; then the domestic animal was harnessed to the wheel and humans could go farther; then the automobile was invented; and now there are modern steamers and air transport. We can draw graphs of man's increased control over space, over time, over manufacture of materials, so that we can make a hundred bolts of cloth in a matter of hours instead of one in a week, and the population can buy as many as they like. That is cumulative: it piles up and piles up; people go faster, make more things, use more materials, and all this is spectacular and exciting.

To see changes in human relationships we have to look inside for changes in pattern. We are not making our changes in human relationships by adding polygamy to monogamy and adding polyandry to polygamy and developing a society which has more forms of marriage; nor are we producing the kind of change of which a graph could be drawn to show monogamy getting more and more intense. If human behaviour be examined on this basis, behind the accumulation of technological change, at the back of all this material and technological progress, is man's consciousness. Man's increasing recognition of the properties of the world around him makes it possible for him to harness power, to breed new kinds of plants and animals, to manufacture by machine rather than by hand, and finally, to make machines which think for him, as we have done since the war.

This increasing understanding has at some point become *self-conscious*. We do not think that the people who invented the wheel knew what they were doing. They were watching something, or starting something, and they developed the wheel, which was the most important invention they knew anything about and they knew it was good. Back in the history of the human race, it took anything from 20,000 to 30,000 years to learn to make a hammer or a knife, which is in contrast to what happens to-day when the laboratory scientist is set a new problem. Thus man has invented invention.

183

When man knew he could invent, it became possible for somebody to say: 'It would be a good thing to have this or that. How shall we make it?'

Looked at in these general terms it can be realized that we are doing the same thing with human relations as we did in the conquest of nature, plants, and elements. We are beginning to see that man can think about himself, that we no longer have to say that whatever peculiar things we do ourselves are natural; that the things other people do are barbarous or peculiar. It is possible to take every detail of our behaviour and subject it to scrutiny, to study the way in which we sit or move, or express the simplest emotion; even to examine why it is that we, here, think it natural to shake the head as a negative, whereas many people will nod their heads instead.

A first step in such a scrutiny would be to consider the peoples of the world as having a common biological inheritance, and then to consider every difference between men as affording information about man's capacity to learn and to change. It may be seen that we have invented invention in the social field in the same way as in a material or mechanical field. The sort of things we are doing in this Seminar are as strange and as new in the world as the sort of things being done in the laboratories of any great concern which is experimenting with new processes or making machines which will think.

One of the dangers we face in attempting to estimate our position is to think of the natural scientist as someone who bends nature to his will, whereas he only proceeds by understanding the laws of nature. Once he has discovered some new law of nature, it is possible for him to work with it, to develop compensatory devices, but nevertheless always to work with it. In our own work we try to do the same thing; we try to discover something about the basic biological laws of human development, so that we can work with them. For example, what can one make of breast-feeding? It was the old view of the natural scientist that it would be an advance to stop breast-feeding entirely. The day-dreams of that period were concerned with the magnificent notion that you might remove a baby from its mother's womb a week after conception and put it in an incubator. A generation was brought up which tried to substitute machinery for inter-personal relations. The whole point of the mental health movement is quite different. We are trying to find out the natural laws and work with them, but it is not sufficient merely to look at the patterns of relationship. To look only at the pattern, as illustrated, for example, by the village, and not at man as a learning animal, is to get only half the story.

If psychiatric services or child development services are looked at in various countries, it can be seen that each country, as it becomes aware of change, develops ways of coping with the first impact of change. It is hard for people to change from country life to city life, to change from one country to another, to give up working with the rhythm of the seasons and work by a clock in a factory: it is hard to substitute self-consciousness for one's intuitive relationship to one's baby, to listen to the public health nurse instead of to the memory of one's grandmother. The public health nurse has become the embodiment of responsible change. The nursery school has replaced the large family; people work in groups to try to overcome their difficulties. As we make these inventions, we can build a new culture of change. The nursery school as compared with the parent is a different medium. One of the necessities of mental health is that there should be a balance between the inside world of the mind and the outside world; if a child with great capacity for imagination is kept in a meagre environment, it will be badly balanced.

Society can change the atmosphere in which different generations of children grow up, in order to prepare them to live flexibly in a changing world and to regard it as their natural environment as a bird regards the winds. We have lived until to-day with a conception of human beings as birds gliding on a still day, with immovable wings, and no capacity to mount on the wings of a gale. Now we know that it is possible to rear human beings who can nest in the gale.

Part Five

SOCIAL AND COMMUNITY
PROVISIONS FOR MENTAL HYGIENE

IMPROVING THE
SOCIAL CARE OF YOUNG CHILDREN
THROUGH PUBLIC HEALTH WORK

Miriam Florentin

PUBLIC HEALTH administration varies from country to country according to the laws of that country and the machinery for central and local government. In England and Wales, during the last ten years there has been major legislation relating to practically all the services in which the Public Health Department is interested. There have been: the Midwives' Act; three Acts relating to adoption; the Children's Act 1948; the Nursery and Child Minders' Act 1948; the National Insurance Act; the National Assistance Act; and the National Health Service Act. In 1944 the new Education Act included an amended statutory basis for the School Health Service, under which the Handicapped Pupils' Regulations have since been made, relating to children from the age of 2. That the country has gone through something of a social revolution can be illustrated from the first two paragraphs of the National Health Service Act:

'It shall be the duty of the Minister of Health . . . to promote the establishment . . . of a comprehensive health service designed to secure improvement in the physical and mental health of the people of England and Wales and the prevention, diagnosis and treatment of illness, and for that purpose to provide or secure the effective provision of services in accordance with the following provisions of this Act.

'The services so provided shall be free of charge, except where any provision of this Act expressly provides for the making and recovery of charges.'

The various parts of the National Health Service Act deal with hospital and specialist health services, services provided by the local health authorities, the general practitioner service, and with social provisions in the mental health services.

On looking at the present public health services in the U.K. in the light of our knowledge of mental health, there appear to be four outstanding needs to be kept in mind:

1. The need to keep the young child with his parents, particularly his mother.

189

2. The need to bear in mind the child's family situation, remembering grandparents, brothers and sisters and the cultural background.
3. The need for knowledge of the normal sequence of development and the factors which influence a child's mental life.
4. A clear appreciation of the need for elasticity in child care.

Our opportunities for education are many, but I think that mental health teaching should permeate all our services, rather than that we should launch an intensive mental health campaign. Among the people to be educated we must include the personnel of the Health Department and those dealing with sick children, young people and parents, and also the administrators, the Town Council, the police and the voluntary organizations. Further research is needed into method, especially into the usefulness of posters, reading, wireless, television and interviews. In our Public Health Departments there are large untapped sources of material relating to the normal child, of which better use should be made in the future, through co-operation of the public health services with psychiatric teams.

It is imperative to ask whether everything possible is done to prepare parents for, and to help them in their task. There is now more talk of preparation for childbirth than of ante-natal care, but do we give enough attention to helping the mother to adjust herself to pregnancy and later to the baby, to understanding the mother's fears and fantasies, and providing for the gaps in her knowledge and her needs? This is particularly true of the unmarried mother. Can anything be done to help the mother, married or unmarried, who is about to give birth to an unwanted baby? What about the unmarried father? Is he never in need of help? One of the British moral welfare associations has recently extended its activities to this field.

On the physical side there is still much to be done. The advice given on diet is still haphazard. Large-scale observations have shown the effect of diet on the still birth, prematurity and neo-natal death rates. According to our records, diet deficiencies can lead to hare lip, cleft palate, and congenital heart disease. Might they not also cause mental deficiency or less obvious abnormalities, and may not various infections in the mother also have effects on the brain and nervous system?

In Britain, fathers now take a much larger share in the care of their children. Could we offer the father evening sessions, with or without his wife, to discuss his problems, and should we run more clubs in connection with our welfare centres? Could we assist the father to make himself more useful in the preparation for and at the

190

time of the confinement? There is an increasing tendency for the husband to be present during the confinement; administering gas and air to his wife is an excellent analgesic for the father! Father does feel excluded from the process of having a baby. Could we not train and employ men in our public health services? There are now a number of male nurses and male home helps and even male nursery nurses.

The decrease in domiciliary confinement is disturbing in some ways, associated as it appears to be in some countries, with episiotomy and low forceps. The Netherlands, with a low maternal mortality have a very good midwifery service with a very high proportion of domiciliary patients. Their maternity aides, who are housekeepers with nursing training, do much to relieve anxiety and keep the family together.

Two disadvantages associated with hospital confinements are the separation of the toddler from his mother, his admission, possibly, to a day-nursery at a most inappropriate moment in his life; and the mother's anxiety about her children's welfare and her husband's doings. We should certainly make available to mothers, opportunities for either home or hospital confinement, and, perhaps, in the absence of definite medical and social indications, she should be the person to choose.

How important is breast-feeding for its own sake? Every nursery nurse can tell the advantages of breast-feeding, but, as an examiner, I sometimes wonder if she will breast-feed her own baby. Many of the physical reasons, except the important one of the transference of immunity, have been discredited; but there may be some other factor not yet discovered. After all, we were unaware of vitamins fifty years ago.

Psychiatric opinion about breast-feeding is not very precise, and is concerned with the baby. It is comfortable to recommend the natural thing, but breast-feeding would hardly seem to come naturally to very many women nowadays. Before we can help to increase the ratio of breast-feeding in the community we need more precision in our knowledge and thinking. Many mothers, for no obvious reason, feel that they cannot or ought not to breast-feed their babies.

Considering the physical environment, housing is very important from the point of view of space, fresh air, safety, and avoidance of friction, and for the provision of such things as laundry services, refuse disposal, and lifts. Outdoor playing space would give the town child something of the advantages of the country child. The housing conditions in some of our cities can be imagined when we realize that there are families in which the mother and children live in one place and the father in another, because of the lack of sleeping space or because they cannot get on with the parents of one of them, with whom they are living. There are a number of families of four living in one room; they sleep, eat, and do everything in the one room, the only means of heat being an open fire and an unguarded gas ring on the floor. The water may have to be carried up, and slops carried down, two or three flights of stairs. It is very important to combat the defeatist attitude which both the public and officials seem to adopt to such housing problems. We cannot afford to postpone good mental health measures until we have achieved good social conditions. There are families who make a reasonably good job of living in conditions such as I have described, and the overcrowding is not worse than before the war. The *Manchester Guardian* recently gave the following figures:

1931: 3.8 per cent of houses had more than two persons living in each room.

1951: 1.4 per cent of houses had more than two persons living in each room.

The collection of facts as proof to reassure parents and officials that children can be brought up, without serious damage, even in these deplorable conditions, would do something to forward the cause of mental health. Observations in Newcastle showed that the mental health of the infant was far more positively dependent on fresh air than negatively on overcrowding. Evidence that a child's development is more closely related to the parents' behaviour than to environmental conditions would give something to work on.

The next point is prevention of accidents. In England and Wales accidental violence is the largest single cause of death among children from 1 to 5 years, the peak age is 2 to 3 and, in addition, many children are maimed for life by accidents in the home. More children are killed by home accidents than on the roads. Some of the safety propaganda makes use of fear, which may be unwholesome for a child brought up to live in a dangerous world. The mother's natural reaction seems to be to give the child a slap or a shaking; this might be a profitable subject for serious study. At what age should the child be taught road sense, and how should it be done?

The time is ripe for a critical review of our routine services for normal children. Should local Health Departments spend less time on routine visits to all infants and children under 5, and more on special visits? Which mothers should be picked out for more intensive visiting—should they be the immature mothers rather than the mothers who are somewhat slipshod housekeepers? Are the common procedures at welfare centres based on a sound conception of physical and mental health? Elimination of much of the routine weighing would relieve mothers of anxiety; most of our standards of normal heights and weights are not only out of date but are based on erroneous conceptions. We need to consider the amount of group technique to employ in educating parents, and which visual aids are appropriate to the subject and audience.

It is an error to concentrate on the baby at the expense of the toddler. There is a risk that babies who are healthy at 12–18 months may develop into under-nourished and debilitated children of 5. There is now a more widespread appreciation of the value of flexibility in infant care. The mother with rigid ideas, who knows that it is abnormal for an older child to suck his thumb, worries because the baby does this very thing. She may be afraid to give the baby night feeds because she thinks that it may establish a habit. In the same way she is afraid to hold the hands of the child who wishes to be comforted as he falls asleep, all because of the lack of appreciation of the normal stages of development.

We all know the mother who says, 'I must begin as I mean to go on.' Similar remarks come from some health visitors, e.g., 'I think the child should not be fed during the night.' But the health visitor who said, 'I teach the mother not to feed the baby during the night, but I think the mothers do feed the babies during the night', and who was not very worried about it, showed greater flexibility.

In planning the future of day-nurseries we must keep a sense of proportion, and though we must avoid damaging the baby there are other people to be considered, particularly the mother. More use might be made of the nurseries for teaching purposes and for rehabilitation of problem families, by letting the mother spend some time in the nursery. Some relief to the constant strain under which mothers live would result from taking children over for short periods. The question of the paid baby-sitter who looks after the children when the parents go out together, needs thought.

In Britain, since 1944, schemes have been developed for the care of premature babies in the home, to include the loan and transport to the home of a cot and other equipment. A recent survey in Newcastle has shown that the mortality among all but the very smallest premature babies nursed at home is less than those who are transferred to hospital.

Space does not allow much discussion of the. schemes for coordination between the hospital, the public health service, and the general practitioner. For handicapped children we now prefer day centres and day care to residential care, and have started a number of such institutions for the care of spastic children, for deaf children and for mentally defective children.

A certain amount of work has been done on problem families,

O   193

both in their own homes and with the help of an institution to which mothers who have been sentenced to prison for neglect of their children can be sent as an alternative to going to prison, and where they are given instruction in child care and housekeeping. A good deal of work has also been done on the education in parentcraft of mothers in prison.

To summarize, there is an immense scope for improvement in the social care of young children through changes within the public health services. To achieve our purpose we may require new legislation or alterations in administrative policy, but much can be done by changing our own approach to our work. We must keep in touch with new knowledge, and be able to apply it with wisdom at the right time. 'Public health is people', and the problems of mental health are a challenge to the people in the public health services.

DISCUSSION

There are some interesting developments in the Netherlands approach to maternity and child care.

In search of improvement, voluntary agencies are establishing health centres in villages, staffed by a nurse, her object being to improve health conditions generally. For a group of villages there is a maternity training centre where a trained nurse teaches young girls living in the region and who come from good families, how to care for lying-in mothers and their babies. The training consists of three months theoretical work with twelve months practical work under supervision, and at the end of fifteen months they are qualified as Maternity Aides. Where the Maternity Aide service is available the still-birth rate is lower than elsewhere, and the death rate of infants in the first week of life is lower. This indicates that simple but professional care by young girls can help the family and thus improve mental health without the word 'mental health' being mentioned.

In the U.K., Home Helps are available during the lying-in period and also in cases of sickness, a service which is organized through the local health authority services, and paid for according to income. The cost of the service sometimes deters the applicants from making use of it.

Some mothers prefer to be in a hospital for a confinement, and feel liberated from the cares of home life, and able to enjoy with the child a certain intimacy which they will never find again. In principle, mothers should be given the opportunity of either domiciliary or hospital confinement. As for the presence of fathers at the confinements, it is of some interest that among the primitive people who, on the whole, are most loved and most highly thought of by Europeans, namely the Polynesians, the father takes an active part in the birth.

A number of British midwives encourage the father to be present, but it needs proper pre-natal education of both father and mother. The midwife would not think of inviting the father to be present unless he and his wife wished it. Those who are in favour say that the labour goes better, the wife is more relaxed, and the practice is something to be encouraged.

In Norway, instead of the term 'illegitimate', the phrase 'born out of wedlock' is used. This reflects the public attitude towards these children, and it is a question whether it helps to improve the emotional atmosphere around such a child to remove the stigma of illegitimacy. Undoubtedly the attitude towards such children is changing in Britain, where a change has been made in the wording of the birth certificate used for everyday purposes, with a view to safeguarding the child.

It still remains to work out how to bring the father more closely into touch with his illegitimate child. The present law in Britain gives the 'illegitimate father' no rights or duties in connection with the child, except that of paying a pittance towards its support on the order of the magistrate.

As regards breast-feeding, one can attach importance to the fact of a woman who can breast-feed her infant refusing to do so: it is almost inevitable that such refusal would lead to a poor emotional relationship with the child and feelings of guilt on the part of the mother.

A policy for homes needs developing, not so much in the belief that overcrowded homes are unhealthy, but that in the kind of society in which we live to-day, a certain independence of life is necessary. Perhaps it is not the size of the home which matters so much as the habits of the family, for if the home is felt as degraded there will be almost inevitable repercussions. People living in caravans as a war measure might adapt quite well to conditions which would have caused a great deal of tension at other times, and the children would react accordingly.

PUBLIC HEALTH SERVICES FOR YOUNG CHILDREN,
ESPECIALLY IN RURAL AREAS

Joyce Akester

MY CONCERN is with Public Health Nursing Services in the U.K. They have grown up in a very haphazard fashion during the past century and in order to understand them, one needs to go back to the Industrial Revolution, and its consequences in the middle of the nineteenth century. An even worse evil than the slums which grew up around the factories was that the young women who left the rural areas came away from their only source of instruction in child care. There were very few books, and the population was still largely illiterate. The children reared in these insanitary conditions, by ignorant mothers, died in thousands.

In 1862 a little group of women in Salford, a neighbouring town to Manchester, formed 'The Ladies' Health Society' and made the first effort to deal with the problems of wastage of child life. They began by delivering leaflets on hygiene and child care, but the leaflets were not read and nothing was done. So they concluded that the only approach was by personal contact and verbal advice. Two 'respectable women' were appointed—we do not even know their names—to teach and advise in the homes on child care, and to distribute soap and disinfectant powder. These two were the first health visitors and this was the beginning of Child Welfare.

Other towns followed the example, and about thirty years later the County Council of Buckinghamshire was the first local government authority to appoint ten Lady Health Missioners. Florence Nightingale took a lively interest in the Buckinghamshire experiment and drew up a course of training for the 'health missioners', as a new profession for women, but there was no suggestion that they should be trained nurses.

In the nineteenth century, midwifery had been a craft passed down from mother to daughter and later in the century the first efforts were made to train midwives; and again Florence Nightingale had a hand in it. At the same time, District Nursing Associations were being formed all over the country, to provide villages and towns with nurses to nurse the sick at home. So by the end of the nineteenth century most of the component parts of the Public Health Nursing Service were already in being.

The first Public Health Act was passed in 1872, under which Medical Officers of Health were appointed, and Milk Stations, the forerunners of Welfare Centres, were established.

In 1902, the Midwives Act made provision for the supervision of midwives and the maintenance of minimum standards of practice. In 1907, the Notification of Births Act paved the way for the full development of the Child Welfare Service by requiring a responsible person to give notice of every birth to the Medical Officer of Health. In 1918, the Maternity and Child Welfare Act, the basis of all child welfare work, gave local authorities power to appoint Medical Officers of Health and Health Visitors; to establish clinics, welfare centres, and day and residential nurseries; to provide free and cheap milk, cod-liver oil, convalescence for mothers and · children, specialist services such as dental and ophthalmic, and many other things. From 1926 all health visitors were required to have nursing and midwifery training, and a special course in health visiting; and from 1936 all Local Authorities have had to maintain a salaried service of midwives, and to provide, free if necessary, a qualified midwife for any woman in childbirth. Lastly, in 1948, the National Health Service Act has included, free of charge, a midwifery, health visiting, and home nursing service.

Meanwhile during the last fifty years the school medical service, the school nursing service and the tuberculosis prevention service have been developed to a high degree.

The situation has been complicated by the option of local authorities either to provide their own services or to pay voluntary organizations to do it for them. The cities have tended to specialize and multiply their own services, whereas in the rural areas, where the work has been delegated to the local voluntary nursing associations, the various functions have been more usually combined in one worker.

Hitherto, the emphasis has been almost entirely on physical health and the prevention of physical illness. Mental health has only found a place in the health visitors' examination syllabus since 1950, and the part that public health nurses can play in the prevention of mental illness is still only being slowly recognized.

Child welfare services in rural areas have developed more slowly than in the towns because the need has been less apparent and less urgent, but most of the usual facilities are now available although, on the whole, they are less easily accessible.

The State provides cheap or free milk, cod-liver oil and orange juice. The milk is delivered by the milkman and cod-liver oil and orange juice have to be fetched from a centre, and in more remote areas are supplied by voluntary workers at distribution stations. Unfortunately only about a third of the mothers take advantage of the scheme, and it is interesting how often mothers will prefer to pay two or three shillings for a proprietary brand of cod-liver oil.

The local health authority provides the domiciliary nursing services, a home-help service, transport to and from hospital by ambulance or car in case of need, vaccination against smallpox, diphtheria and other immunization, welfare centres and clinics, including such special clinics as child guidance, ophthalmic, orthopaedic, dental, speech therapy, etc. Day-nurseries, which are included in city child welfare schemes, are not commonly found in rural areas, because of insufficient demand.

The special clinics are usually established in the local towns, so that country children may have a long bus journey, sometimes with an infrequent service. Welfare centres have been developed in big villages, but since they meet only once a week or once a month they have to be held in church or village halls which are not always as suitable as we would wish and, because of lack of storage space, health education materials have to be kept to a minimum. In spite of these disadvantages the weekly or fortnightly sessions are generally very well attended. In the small villages with a very few inhabitants there are 'Weighing Centres', (though 'Advice Centre' would be a better name) attended by the health visitor alone. She has foods available, weighs the children and advises the mothers, or, if necessary, recommends that a child be taken to its general practitioner. In the larger villages, a doctor may be in attendance once a month, and in some counties 'travelling clinics' serve the scattered population of remote villages and hamlets.

Country mothers appreciate the companionship and conversation of the welfare centre, and their visits may not be solely for the purpose of having babies weighed, receiving advice and obtaining cod-liver oil. This is a time to discuss knitting patterns over cups of tea and to exchange recipes, while their children rush about in the waiting-room playing with their toys. Such a setting gives the health visitor a very good opportunity for unrehearsed health education, and at the same time, it meets a need of these children who live in remote cottages and have no other chance of meeting children of their own age. In the villages also, where the cinema is less accessible, a film is always appreciated, and the mothers will discuss it afterwards. Village mothers like to have exhibitions of home made garments and competitions in toymaking, cookery, etc. Mothers' Clubs have sometimes grown out of welfare centres, and the mothers' knowledge can be used for the benefit of friends and neighbours with less ability.

But in the country, even more than in the towns, the value of the child welfare service depends ultimately on its medical and public health nursing officers. There is constant need and scope for the use of imagination and initiative, and the ability to improvise.

Some counties have a staff of assistant medical officers who attend the welfare centres, and who are specially qualified in public health and child care. Other authorities employ general practitioners on a part-time basis, but often the latter have not been trained in preventive medicine, and may have little interest in either the mental or the physical development of the normal healthy child. Moreover this practice becomes complicated when the village is served by more than one doctor.

In the country areas the public health nurse usually has the function either of the district-nurse/midwife/health visitor in one, sometimes called the generalized public health nurse—or there is a district-nurse/midwife and a health visitor.

In a sparsely populated area the generalized public health nurse provides the most economical type of service. The nurse lives in the village and conducts a surgery for minor ailments; she is very often guide, counsellor and friend and, especially if there is no doctor in the village, she is the first person to be called in any crisis or emergency.

The good country nurse must be able to find her own interests and to live contentedly within the limited circle of the village. She is almost perpetually on call, except for her one day off a week. She must also be prepared for all the hardships of life in the country in the winter, and her nights are often disturbed. No other nurse in the public health service needs a stronger sense of vocation.

The greatest disadvantage of generalized work is the tendency for prevention to be sacrificed to cure, whenever there is pressure of work, and there is also a natural tendency for nurses to concentrate on one side of their work at the expense of the others. To meet these disadvantages, many authorities use two types of worker—the district-nurse/midwife and the health visitor. This means that there may be some overlapping. The health visitor has to travel long distances, is not readily available locally, and is often not able to visit frequently. Meanwhile the district-nurse is called for all the minor crises—teething difficulties, vomiting, and so on. Country people accept the district-nurse more readily than the health visitor.

Against these disadvantages must be set the great advantage that both the health visitor and the nurse/midwife are doing the work of their choice. The approach of the health visitor to her work differs from that of the sick nurse. The health visitor discerns and attempts to meet different needs, so that the mothers who seek the advice of the district-nurse for a skin rash will save their problems of child

199

behaviour or family relationships for the health visitor. On the whole, rural authorities favour the dual method of staffing, and with good co-operation between the nurse/midwife and the health visitor it works reasonably well.

At the present time, the physical health and development of children in Britain is quite good, except for some black spots, but other problems still unsolved include:

How to improve the homes and prospects of these children;

How co-operation between family doctors and local authorities can be increased;

How the family doctors who attend welfare centres can play their full part in preventing physical and mental ill-health;

What type of public health nursing service is the best in rural areas;

How the health visitor of the future should be trained: is there a case for a different type of training?

How her work can be designed in order not to overlap with that of other social workers;

How in-service training in mental health can be given to public health nurses;

How mental health can be integrated into the nurse's general and public health training.

These and many other unanswered questions give much food for thought. We are very conscious of shortcomings in our present service, but when we look at our records and at our children we take pride in the achievements of the past and have confidence in the future.

DISCUSSION

Possibly an unduly pessimistic view has been taken about the relationship between the general practitioner and the health visitor.

The fault lies with those who teach medical students only in the artificial surroundings of wards and out-patients' departments, and who fail to give them any concept of the emotional, economic and social factors in the home. In some medical schools, now, each medical student is given a family to follow right through his course.

In Australia in the remote waste tracts, the 'flying doctor' with his own plane is based on a small country hospital with two or three nurses, and all the people have radio sets. The doctor represents a happy combination of the practising surgeon, physician, and public health officer. There are six doctors, each responsible for a 500-mile radius, and each of the big farmhouses has its own radio transmitter and can call at certain periods during the day for urgent help, or get advice about the use of the medicine chest in the house. Either a doctor or a sister might go out to the case or the patient might be brought into the hospital. A start has now been made to arrange welfare centres in the same way, and there is also a system by which the children in their homesteads can get answers to their questions by wireless from the school.

In general, however, in respect of mental hygiene, many doctors and even the personnel of Maternity and Child Welfare Departments still do not have much interest in the community but are interested only in the cure of disease.

The child care services in the United Kingdom have been in a rather changed situation since 1948. An unfortunate death by neglect of a foster child brought about a national uproar, and a Government Committee of Inquiry advised that the care of such children should be centralized under one department instead of being divided between the health, education, and public assistance authorities. Eventually it became administratively expedient to make the Home Office the central authority for 'deprived' children. New local 'Children's Departments' have been formed to look after all the children who are deprived of normal home life. Many of the new officials hold some qualification in social science but are not necessarily experienced in the care of children, and their quality is variable.

A new form of training has been improvised for the new 'children's visitors', whose background is even more variable, and some have had no training at all. Inevitably tensions have arisen between the public health departments and the new children's departments, and health visitors naturally are inclined to see in the children's visitor an encroachment upon their work; but in spite of this, an effort is being made to establish good co-operation between the two departments.

Child welfare work, however, is something of a battlefield in the U.K. General practitioners have suffered criticism because of their general lack of interest in preventive work, but many of them who work in country districts consider, not without justification, that, having lived in the district all their lives, they know the people. They recall having not only delivered the present child, but the child's mother and father. They are sometimes inclined to regard the district-nurse, and the children's visitor also, for that matter, in those cases where the mutual relationship is not so good, as rather an officious person, not always very wise in handling people.

When people have to devote their lives to the care of other people's children, they live under great strain. Some of the district midwives in country districts have been living for a very long time under such a strain; they have brought other people's babies into the world for a generation, but this does not always mean that they can handle family problems.

Sometimes there are the most happy relationships, even amongst the general practitioners and the health visitors in a town, where the antagonism perhaps tends to be deeper-rooted.

The question as to who is encroaching on whose territory is extremely controversial. For example, many of the social workers maintain that they have been in the field since before health visitors or even district-nurses became general; though it is true that the first Health Visitors' Society predated the first social service voluntary organization by about twenty years. In Britain social workers have engaged in family case-work for about two generations, whereas health visitors have not been trained specifically in case-work up to now. They have often had to do it, but without the necessary preparation.

Little instruction in mental hygiene is included in the basic nursing training, and the little psychology which has been included has been of a rather academic type and restricted to six lectures only. Since 1950 some mental health training has been included in the health visitors' syllabus: before that they were taught to look upon the child simply as a body unencumbered by a mind and a soul.

However, nurses in training are not necessarily bound by what is officially in the syllabus. Many keep their eyes and ears and minds wide open and are receptive to ideas now prevalent in mental hygiene teaching. The history of the development of their work with the normal child justifies the feeling of public health nurses that they are being passed over.

For example, their ante-natal work has been so successful that the obstetricians have taken it over, which was fair enough. Then preventive child health proved so successful that the paediatricians took it over; now they have to watch the psychiatrists taking over the mental health of the well child. Their view is that the physical, the mental, and the emotional aspects of the very young are so closely integrated that anyone supervising the normal child must have an understanding of all three.

Experience as a maternity and child welfare officer, and also as a general practitioner, might suggest that in future the general practitioner should undertake the clinical part of preventive medicine, when properly trained in the preventive aspect of the work and in paediatrics, and when he is willing to work as a member of a team and to keep records.

The curative side, which is going to get less, needs to be very closely integrated with the preventive service; but in Britain, the National Health Service has, unfortunately, split up the health services for children between general practice, the hospital service and the local authority service. Having been split up they must now be put together again.

In the United States and Great Britain in particular, administrators are always cutting things up and then having a liaison committee to put them together again. In every city of the United States there are separately organized series of family agencies and children's agencies, and when they have to have a merger it is painful for all the people deeply concerned in the work.

With this sort of experience it is disheartening to learn how the recent National Health Service Act in Britain has done a new piece of cutting up. It is conceivable that those countries in which nationwide health services are very young might avoid some of these errors, by keeping their eye on whole issues. Then they will not have three or four services, one dealing with the mind of the child, another with its body, and a third with its soul: if they also think about the mother and the child together, they will get further, and if they think about the whole family they will get even more unification.

The notion that the mother and child is the most important unit, leaves out fathers. If all the members of the family are considered all the time, when they are sick and well, at home and away, it becomes impossible to split up services. A great many clues are supplied by good rural services: perhaps the Australian is the most striking, because in the rural areas it is necessary to work with people where they live and not to take them away.

Another danger is that services will be organized in other, less developed, parts of the world by people familiar with such developments as have been described, with the result that in some far distant country there might be reproduced on a considerable scale techniques common in the United States or Britain some years ago, but now in process of change.

COMMUNITY ACTION TO IMPROVE
THE CONDITIONS OF LIFE OF
THE YOUNG CHILD

Alan A. Moncrieff

MY TASK is to open a discussion on the part that the community should play to ensure satisfactory conditions of life for the normal or average child in the normal or average home and on what the community can do to help such a child. I want to stress particularly the physical side, of which we have more experience, and perhaps we can learn from our mistakes and successes in that field what to do on the psychological side, which is much more difficult from the community point of view.

We would all agree that it is the duty of the community to provide safe and satisfactory environmental conditions for the young child; that is, it is the duty of the community to provide a safe water supply, to be concerned with drains, with satisfactory housing, to prevent nuisances, overcrowding, and things of that sort. We should also pay attention as a community to the safety of children in houses, schools and streets. With the great improvement in physical health in this country, the greatest menace to the child after the first year of life is not the microbe but the motor car. Far more children nowadays die as a result of accidents than as a result of disease, so that it is a community duty to see that care is taken to prevent accidents both in the home and the street. It is a community duty to safeguard children with regard to their food; to lay down standards and enforce them, to ensure that the food supply is good. But here is a point of controversy: there is, in the provision of a safe food supply, a hint of interference with the liberty of the individual. For example, talk about safe milk in this country rouses the antagonism of the farmers and others, who say that they are not concerned with the safety of milk but that people should get fresh milk straight from the farms. It is important for a community wanting to take action which it thinks is good, to take note of matters resented by groups within it.

The community can and should take action with regard to the control of communicable diseases. The prevention of typhoid fever, for example, is a question of a safe water supply. Other means include regulations concerning the provision and sale of certain foods, and of preventive inoculation and vaccination. Once more we reach the problem of whether such inoculations and vaccinations should be compulsory or not. Up to 1948 vaccination against smallpox was compulsory in the United Kingdom, but it was resisted by a large number of people who regarded it as interference with their individual freedom. There was introduced many years ago what was called the 'conscientious objection clause', by which a person, or in the case of an infant, a parent, could make a declaration that they had a conscientious objection to vaccination. Sixty to 75 per cent of parents had been contracting out in this way, for Great Britain is the happy hunting-ground of people who are 'anti-everything'.

The campaign for voluntary inoculation against diphtheria has been so successful that 70 to 80 per cent of children have been inoculated under four or five years of age. It was, therefore, decided to abolish compulsion in regard to smallpox vaccination; but it would take an outbreak of smallpox to frighten people into having their children vaccinated. When should a community take compulsory powers in matters of this kind? At what stage of a problem is a community sufficiently affected to accept compulsory powers? Much depends on the incidence of a disease within the country: if slight, it is difficult to persuade people of the importance of inoculation, and this is the position in Britain over the limited voluntary inoculation with B.C.G. against tuberculosis with which we are cautiously feeling our way.

With some diseases, prevention can be a more personal matter, unlike the safeguarding of a water supply which is a community action. A particular disease, affecting a particular child, may set a personal problem which has to be tackled in a very different way. First, there is the whole field of health education, effected most commonly by means of pamphlets, books and posters, films, newspaper propaganda and broadcasting. The community obviously can play a part in this, either directly or indirectly. In Britain, perhaps, a Government publication may not be as successful as a pamphlet sponsored by some non-governmental body.

The most successful health education in Britain of recent years has been that put out by the Radio Doctor. Mothers listened to what he said and carried it out to a greater degree than anything achieved by any other method. All depends upon the personality of the speaker, his material, how it is put across and so on. This successful measure, contrary to popular belief, was not Government-sponsored.

More specific health education in relation to the young child must be undertaken mainly through the welfare centres and the school health services. Is the right way to have a talk with mothers during or after their visits to the clinic? Is it better to give them something to read? Or is it better to try to tackle them individually? Is it better to try to make parents do things for themselves?

An interesting experiment was made recently in Buckinghamshire, where in quite small village areas considerable success in health education was achieved by giving groups of parents a particular task to do. It was decided to hold an exhibition and during the winter months the groups were asked to make the material for an exhibition which was aimed at explaining the improvement in living conditions during the last hundred years. One group dealt with clothing, another with a safe milk supply, another with housing and so on. These mothers and fathers produced an exhibition which they all saw, prizes being given for the best exhibit. To make their exhibits they had to study their subject, and the whole project was a good example of learning by doing. Every one of the parents who helped to make the exhibition would always remember its lesson. At child welfare and school health centres, health education should be part of the general curriculum; and the school medical officer should himself help in the schools in the general health education programme.

The deficiency diseases illustrate different problems in preventive medicine. First, rickets: the late Sir Gowland Hopkins discovered the cause of rickets before the First World War; other workers added to the knowledge, and about 1919 Sir Edward Mellanby showed conclusively that rickets could be produced in puppies by depriving them of vitamin D and that the condition could be cured by cod-liver oil. In 1939 rickets still existed in the country in spite of efforts to persuade mothers to use cod-liver oil, which was on sale. Later it was provided free, but never more than 30 per cent of mothers attending welfare clinics took it, and some of these mothers used it for purposes other than that intended—such as polishing furniture—so we cannot tell the degree of its use for children.

Three important decisions were made at the beginning of the 1939–45 war: vitamin D was added to margarine, the basic fat available, and to all dried milk. No baby could now avoid getting an adequate quantity of vitamin D: if he was breast-fed he got it from his mother's margarine, and if he was bottle-fed he got it in the dried milk food. So, by community action, rickets has virtually disappeared.

Secondly, if there is adequate fluorine in the water supply there is less dental caries: in certain areas in Britain a much lower rate of dental caries has been correlated fairly definitely with the amount of fluorine in the water. But the suggestion that in those areas where the amount of fluorine in the water was not adequate, some should be added to the reservoirs, has been strongly resisted in many quarters.

Thirdly, because of a lack of calcium in the wartime dietary, calcium was added to bread. This practice also has been attacked by bodies such as the British Housewives' League, one of whose slogans relates to fresh food which has not been 'adulterated'. The choice of this word is subtle, because it implies shame. No one who believes in reinforcing food would care to say, 'I believe in adulteration of food', so this very clever piece of propaganda immediately disarms the critics. The Housewives' League protests against fluorine being added to water as well as against the addition of calcium to bread, and it is probably only a matter of time before they become aware of the fact that vitamin D is added to margarine and dried milk.

We have learned as a community how to prevent rickets and several other diseases, yet there still exist public bodies which say that the community has no right to compel such action to prevent disease, that people must be left to choose for themselves the sort of food they require, that the Government and the community must neither alter nor reinforce the food available nor 'adulterate' it. Is the community justified in restricting freedom of choice so as to make it impossible for any mother in England to buy dried milk without the addition of vitamin D? Unfortunately the argument that there was vitamin D in the milk before the process of drying destroyed it, and that we have only put it back, is quite ineffective.

The provision of safe milk by community action has also been criticized. It has been difficult to persuade people to have pasteurized milk, because of a popular belief that when milk is pasteurized it loses all its vitality and that 'all the good has gone out of it'. During the war, as an economy measure, the distribution of milk was zoned so that, for example, there should be only one source of supply to one street. Since this would force some people to buy unsafe milk, the Government tried to secure that all milk was pasteurized. By a curious paradox therefore, by abolishing free choice of milk, far more milk was pasteurized than ever before. It is still possible to buy unsafe milk if one wishes to, but the standard of milk has been gradually raised as the necessary machinery and skill have become available. This community action was criticized as taking away liberty of choice, but it will prevent a great deal of disease.

How far is compulsion justified, not only in regard to the prevention of communicable diseases or to food, but in regard to the removal of infected patients? In Britain, only in a case of smallpox can we compel a patient to go to hospital. A person can lie at home with active, open, tuberculosis and infect his whole family and no one has the power to remove him. I once conspired with a tuberculosis officer in the removal to a sanatorium of a tuberculous mother of a family of young children. We had no power to override her refusal to go, but we applied such sanctions as refusing books from the public library and forbidding the supply of milk in bottles, and eventually she was glad to go. But we have no direct power to remove a person who is suffering from infectious disease. To what extent should we apply compulsion if the health of a young child is suffering by contact? In the long run, of course, it would be ideal to educate the public so that they would demand the application of compulsion, but this, in this country particularly, may take a very long time.

Community action in regard to psychological matters is much more difficult still, partly because there is much less experience, except of course in the successful experiment of compulsory education. But what can the community do in seeking to prevent the more specific psychological troubles, and to provide the psychological environment in which children can best grow up? It can give the parents badly needed education in the more subtle and only recently understood matters of child development.

Bowlby's report on Maternal Care and Mental Health (2) draws attention to what he called the 'vitamins of mental health', education and security. This is a very useful phrase, for these so-called 'vitamins' are essential for the full development of the young child. But besides filling the obvious needs, the community has a responsibility to prevent cruelty, both physical and psychological—what might be called the police function of the community. This is a somewhat difficult function, for it means a certain amount of interference with personal liberty. There are in Britain to-day far too many people with power to interfere with the natural home and to remove children to what they may consider to be better circumstances. As a community we have to try to help parents bring up their children at home even in cases of physical or psychological illness. We shall have to consider how children who are likely to be ill for a long time can receive care and education in their homes, rather than in hospitals, schools, and so on. We have to make more attempts to deal with acutely sick children in their own homes, in the light of modern thought on the subject of the separation of very young children from their parents. Our slogan should be, 'Keep children out of hospital except as a last resort.'

The community, in planning for children deprived of normal home care, must favour the fostering of children in small groups, boarding them out with foster parents, and breaking up large children's institutions into cottage homes and families. This subject is still controversial, but it is the policy in favour with the community in this country at the present time. Also, in the training of staff, the importance is emphasized of the small imitation family for children who have no family of their own.

The community, then, has a duty to educate parents with regard to the best type of parent-child relationship; it has the duty of teaching preventive mental hygiene and this has mainly to be done through the existing machinery of welfare centre and school health service. I think we have to remind parents that their children are not chattels about whom they can boast as if they were personal property, but that they are human souls to hold in trust during the period of development and maturation. We have to teach parents elementary things of this sort, that the child has constantly to be encouraged in its move towards independence, that the more the child can develop its independence the more it will develop its character and the more real will be the bonds of affection with its parents.

When parents have neglected their children it is futile to punish them by sending them to prison. The community's job is, surely, to try to educate them towards a better understanding of their children's needs. In all these things we are groping our way towards the best methods of achieving, in a practical manner, these aims of preventive mental hygiene.

DISCUSSION

The Radio Doctor is not sponsored either by the Government or the paediatricians. The holder of this appointment is engaged direct by the British Broadcasting Corporation. The first Radio Doctor had a way of expressing things which, though disliked by some people, put across health matters in a way never before achieved. He stimulated questions and answered many that mothers had not been able to formulate to their own welfare centres and clinics.

The B.B.C. is an independent Corporation, and although occasionally Government officials ask for some particular broadcast to be made—for instance, the Chief Medical Officer of the Ministry of Health has broadcast on vaccination and on venereal diseases—normally health education is a part of the B.B.C.'s own programme.

Radio has had a powerful effect in breaking down verbal taboos: people can now talk about health and disease using direct words in a way they could not have done even ten years ago.

It is of interest to review conditions in other countries in regard to compulsory inoculation.

Smallpox vaccination is compulsory in Egypt; it is accepted by the people and carried out in the first three months after birth.

In Yugoslavia, vaccination against smallpox is obligatory; and the people have become accustomed to the annual visit of the doctor to the villages, to carry out the vaccinations, and thus contact is made between the doctor and the people, which is a good thing from the point of view of health education and is one of the benefits, in a backward country, of accepting compulsory vaccination. Also in Yugoslavia inoculation against diphtheria and B.C.G. vaccination after the age of 1 year, are obligatory; and these have contributed to education in hygiene.

This represents a great advance; however, it should be remembered that the child has no choice in the matter, and he is the person most affected. Freedom of choice for the parent might be almost an irrelevant consideration in this issue.

In Belgium, vaccination against smallpox is compulsory, while inoculation against diphtheria is widespread but not compulsory.

In political dependencies there is a particular danger of changes in public opinion becoming identified with political attitudes. In French North Africa and Algeria, vaccination has been generally well accepted and during the past two years B.C.G. vaccination has been introduced by mobile medical units in the villages. During the war, political factions put out propaganda against vaccination, saying that it was being used by the French to reduce the native population, and in this way a considerable resistance to vaccination was built up.

In Switzerland, vaccination before school age is compulsory for diphtheria and smallpox. With regard to B.C.G. vaccination, a campaign advocating voluntary protection of children against tuberculosis has been organized, with a large measure of success.

In Sweden it is held that health measures should be compulsory, but backed with propaganda so that people may know why they are compelled to carry them out. Vaccination against smallpox is compulsory, and B.C.G. vaccination against tuberculosis is widespread but not compulsory, being a subject of propaganda by school doctors and others. The children are used to educate the parents. In Stockholm dental caries had been very much on the increase, so the school authorities sent to the parents, by the small children, a letter surrounded with flowers which they could paint. Inside there was a letter written by the child to its mother: 'My teacher has told me about eating sweets, that it is not good for my teeth, and I ask you not to give me so many sweets.' The children and the teacher talked about the effects of eating sweets, and when the child took the letter home to the parents it had a very good effect.

In Germany there is compulsory vaccination against smallpox, but not in the first year. It is hoped by propaganda to encourage parents to have the vaccination carried out at an earlier age in order to avoid the risk of encephalitis. Voluntary inoculation against diphtheria has included 80 per cent of the children, but inoculation against tuberculosis is not so popular, and depends very much on the doctors in the neighbourhood.

It is very noticeable that when there is an outbreak of smallpox in Britain the rush for vaccination is quite phenomenal. In one village where all the children under 5 were vaccinated, the deaths of a few distant fellow-countrymen had done far more than years of persuasion and education. This raises the controversial issue of the introduction of a little more wholesome fear into the propaganda.

However, in a number of campaigns in the United States, notably the cancer and the poliomyelitis campaigns, a certain amount of uneasiness and guilt have been produced by the kind of literature which was disseminated. The kind of advertising propaganda used to get women and older people especially, to go to so-called cancer clinics for examination, may generate such fear about these diseases that an extra burden is thrown on the general practitioner and on the specialist in these clinics, beyond their powers to bear, and this has repercussions on the campaign.

Another interesting effect in the U.S.A., in relation to poliomyelitis, has been the selling of insurance policies against the disease, which has made at least one Company's fortune. This question of 'wholesome fear' is a delicate one; there may be repercussions from propaganda or health education on the incidence of mental illness. Health propaganda in the U.S.A. does not commonly give relatively constructive hints on health. Obviously propaganda must be suitable for the cultural background of the country in which it is put forward.

Wholesome fear, which has been mentioned, is fear of something that one dislikes, and about which something can be done. It is not wholesome to make people afraid of something about which nothing can be done. In this sense there is a place for 'wholesome fear' in health education.

People remember best what they can laugh at—a fact well recognized by commercial firms in advertising; but health education experts are inclined to think that their subject is too serious to make jokes about.

There has been compulsory vaccination in France for a long time, but it is necessary to support compulsion by propaganda to get results. Propaganda for vaccination must be efficient, and radio can now play an important part, but only if the material is presented in an assimilable form.

Until this year there has been compulsory vaccination in Finland. Its abolition seems to have been because of the delicate political situation and the people's sensitivity about freedom. It was thought that they could get along without any compulsion. Other vaccination is voluntary, but on the other hand, patients with dangerous in-fective illnesses are removed compulsorily to hospitals.

In Denmark vaccination against smallpox is compulsory, although some people oppose it. Inoculation against diphtheria is not compulsory but the children are not admitted to nursery schools without it. B.C.G. vaccination is given to all children beginning school and there is a campaign to give it to children leaving school. It is now also being offered to all children born in hospitals and clinics.

The question of compulsory vaccination should concern all democratic countries. Should people be allowed to run the risk of doing harm to others? If a parent does not have a child vaccinated there is the risk of an epidemic. It would be difficult to deal with an epidemic of leprosy in Europe nowadays because few countries have powers to segregate lepers, and this lack of power makes for difficulties in the prevention of tuberculosis. *A priori* it might be argued that one should not allow diseases to propagate any more than one should tolerate murder.

It may be beneficial to divert the argument away from any question of policy *versus* freedom. For example, in one State in America, with endemic goitre among the population, about twenty years ago, iodine was added to the salt; the salt-makers were persuaded to put it in and people knew it was good. Twenty years later it was discovered that the iodine had disappeared from the salt because the awareness of its necessity had vanished. Safeguards must be taken so that such practices do not die away. For instance, one might make a rule that no child could be admitted to school without a vaccination certificate: this would create a pattern of practice which could be reinforced by the public authorities in order to get people to do what they ought to do. Without such patterns, the educational work would be interminable.

There has not been much resistance in the U.S.A. to reinforced food. Americans love a bargain, and the more there is in the bread the better. There is resistance in California, however, to the inclusion of fluorine in the water. When the Health Department recommended it a number of communities voted acceptance, but there was resistance from two groups, one a religious movement which believes that fluorine is medicine and contrary to their beliefs; and another which feels that the addition of a chemical to the water supply is an invasion of their public rights. Although the groups were very much in the minority the programme was held up until the Attorney-General decided that the State Department was within its rights.

One of the most striking and serious examples of the way in which a minority could hold the rest of the community to ransom was exhibited at the World Health Assembly of 1952, at which a request that WHO should, in the interests of the starving peoples of over-populated areas, discuss the question of birth control, was refused because a minority group would not allow it even to be discussed, hinting at possible withdrawal from the Organization.

Day and residential nurseries are sometimes justified on the grounds that children can go there for certain features of their up-bringing and that mothers can be taught there to care for their children. The main question is whether the educational value of a day-nursery will offset the disadvantage to the child of being separated from his mother at that age. The answer may well be a matter of choosing the lesser evil. If a mother has to go to work, the child may be better off in a properly-run nursery than in the care of a neighbour. If the mother can provide a good home background it is not good for the child to be taken away from its mother each day and supervised by other people.

The rights of parents in relation to their sick children is a burning topic in Britain at present, particularly the question of visiting sick children in hospital, the care of babies by their own mothers in hospital, the extension of home nursing for sick children, and the role of the paediatrician in the first few weeks of life.

It is too early to say anything about home nursing of sick children, but there are one or two centres in Britain which hope to experiment in the hospital nursing of sick children in their own homes. Child-ren's Hospitals are changing their attitude to the visiting of parents and to the use of parents, particularly mothers, in the care of their children in hospital. For many years children's hospital work has been dominated by the fear of infection, for it is a serious matter if a child goes in for a routine operation and contracts another infec-tion. Until hospitals have buildings with facilities for isolation, and abolish the large open ward unit, and employ adequate numbers of nursing staff, this fear of infection is justified. There is no positive statistical evidence that visiting has anything to do with cross in-fection. The incidence of infection is not related to whether children are freely visited or not. Having established this, hospitals are much more free to experiment with the visiting of children by their parents, encouraged by the work of Bowlby and others.

Many Children's Hospitals have now established daily visiting by mothers, and this policy is officially encouraged. Every mother who lives near enough is encouraged to come every day between five and six to put her child to bed at night, doing the same things for the child as if it were at home, bathing it and giving it supper, reading to it, saying prayers, and waiting until it is asleep. This is a helpful way of maintaining the child's contact with its mother. He can remember her when he wakes and he can just about hold out for the rest of the day until she comes again. If the mother cannot come every day perhaps a neighbour will do so and that is quite acceptable. There is room for cautious experiment with fathers. Little girls miss their fathers very much. In some places the experiment is very much liked by the nurses, and it is very good for them to see more of the mother-child relationship.

In the case of very young babies, the need is to minimize the number of faces which the small baby sees. This can be done by case assignment, as far as possible to one or two or three nurses, so that the baby is not completely baffled by complexity.

The mother can play a part in the nursing of her child, though a sick child requires a great deal of technical help which the mother cannot necessarily give. When the child is seriously ill the mother is no more than an amateur. For example, one of the most needful things for a febrile child is an adequate intake of fluid, and mothers are not as good as the professional nurse in getting fluid into a child. Apart from this it is a good thing for the mother to be about as much as possible, to come to the hospital and take over from the nursing staff for some days before the baby goes home, so that the baby going out from hospital does not find its own mother a complete stranger.

MENTAL HYGIENE AND THE CARE OF CHILDREN UNDER CONDITIONS OF FAMILY OR SOCIAL CHANGE

Kent A. Zimmerman

MY TASK is to examine in a general way how community agencies can apply the principles of mental hygiene in the care of the child. Perhaps the first need is to apply increasingly the concept of the principles of growth and development, and of relationships, to the practice in institutions and then, later, to take community factors into account.

At present those who are engaged in the practical application of the principles of mental hygiene work on their own, using intuition, knowledge and their own point of view in each new situation. In an attempt to get more systematic order into guiding principles, we might briefly examine first, the principles of emotional growth and development, breaking them down and then re-examining them in terms of application to institutions. First I should like to define our terms. 'Mental hygiene', as used here, means those techniques, and their application to individuals and institutions, used in order to attain a better state of mental health. 'Mental health', in a very broad sense, might be defined as the goal of our attempts to achieve for each individual the development of his potential capacities so that he will be respected by himself and by the groups of which he is a member. That does not imply conformity to all situations because, as we have found out, even a child may find that it is better for his own self-respect not to conform to some situations.

I would like to review what I have learned from case histories prepared for the Seminar, in terms of thought now popular in the United States. At the last White House Conference in the United States (held every ten years to examine and review the programmes for children and also to plan for the future) the emphasis was on a healthy personality for every child. One of the important contributions was that of Dr. Eric Erikson whose book entitled, *Childhood and Society* (9) embodies some of his ideas, based on a Freudian or dynamic concept of growth and development. It is amazing how rapidly people, not in the field of psychiatry, have become able to use concepts of human relationships to which, hitherto, they have been somewhat resistant. These concepts are, currently, a means of good communication in a very technical field. At the Conference, when more orthodox technical analytic terms were used, no great effect was obtained, whereas when Erikson formulated his concepts in basic English, people felt that now, somebody was 'talking for me, too'.

The primary fact to be gathered from the Seminar case studies is that a baby has a past—a learning past—learning from his parents, as rapidly as possible, what the world is like. He has to learn what he needs for his survival and growth, and in so doing, a two-way communication is established. For instance, it has been said that the first response of a child to his parents is his smile, which comes at 3 or 4 months. But I think we have learnt that a mother in the early weeks has come to feel the need of the biological response of the infant. She takes note of his physical condition, whether his bowels are moving, whether he vomits or not, and she interprets these in a very personal way and gets response from the infant in return.

The Seminar histories show again, the importance of heredity and constitution; but beyond that they show that it is important to think of the infant as sensitive to the mother person; and even more than this, case examples show that when the mother's true feelings for her child were inhibited, the child responded in a much more psychologically pathological way.

Baby health seems to depend on how well the baby learns his lesson, of which the first is to learn from his environment how to obtain and accept what is given him. This he learns through the methods devised by his culture as well as by his mother. By these early steps, the baby learns to become a giver also. Consistency in the attitude of his parents, especially his mother, towards him and consistency in the satisfaction of his biological needs are essential to this learning. We have come to recognize that inconsistency in maternal behaviour (and absence of the mother or maternal figure is one variety of inconsistency), has adverse effects. But more subtly, and more important, we now recognize that inconsistency will come most from parents who have inhibited feelings of resentment, hostility, and anger about the child, disguised from themselves. The experience by the baby of this fact and the receipt of this communication lead to signs of stress. Continued inconsistency of maternal behaviour and of maternal communication seems to lead to the child's basic sense of mistrust, which is a much more pathological reaction.

I think we have learned from 'rooming-in',[1] and especially from the case histories in relation to pregnancies, that the basic sense of

[1] See 'Child Development Patterns in the U.S.A.', Jackson, p. 87.

trust and the beginnings of healthy maternal communication depend upon the mother working through the normal psychological problems of her pregnancy. These problems consist usually of her attitude about dependency and perhaps the clarification of her own role as a mother, especially in relation to her identification with her own mother. In the U.S. we can see the working out of this psychological problem when the mother leaves the maternity ward of the hospital and takes the baby home. She often experiences for the first few days an emotional reaction known as the 'Going home blues', a mild depression when faced with her own dependence. The mother is encouraged in a dependent relationship by institutional practice and by her relationship with the obstetrician. After the coming of the baby this must quickly change, but in hospital, baby and mother had little time to spend together and it is only later that the mother is faced with the prospect of taking sole charge of the infant herself on the day she goes home. She goes back home, where perhaps her own mother has come to help her, thereby re-awakening any old mother-daughter relationship problems. In this situation she needs support and help.

In the first six months after the baby's arrival the influence of the father becomes somewhat removed, but he influences the mother; and certainly his ability or otherwise to share the satisfaction of his own needs in his home with the close attention that has now to be given to the young child is important to the family adjustment.

These matters are important to administrators and professional persons, because, in principle, they should have a scientific basis for their activities and plans so that they may be independent of the attitude or prestige of people trying to get them to make changes. For example, a study was done in a hospital some years ago on crying occurring in a new-born babies' nursery and how it could be reduced. It was found that the amount of crying could be reduced by about half if one-third more nursing staff were added. Some hospital administrators, however, said, 'Why do this? It is expensive to add nurses or to train aides. Even if the baby cries, he will soon be taken out of hospital and the mother will have him.' But the basis on which to examine such a problem is to know whether the baby requires to begin to learn something important to him from a maternal figure even during its first few days in hospital—a period at times of ten days.

Let us consider more carefully the lessons to be learnt from 'rooming-in'. The usual care given to the pregnant woman, in other than primitive communities, has certain basic patterns. First, the woman relies on the obstetrician or midwife for her security and for working through her normal psychological problems of pregnancy.

When a woman has to relate herself to an institution for her delivery more than to an individual doctor or midwife, new manœuvres must be introduced to provide this security. To this end, instruction classes for pregnant women are often organized and led by nurses, and the mothers obtain support from them in this teaching relationship but probably more so from each other, as all face similar problems.

Secondly, the practices of institutions change within a very few years. For example, recently in the United States, the President's Commission on the Health Needs of the Nation, explored new problems with regard to children. The obstetric consultant brought figures to prove that, taking into account the increasing number of births and the number of obstetricians available, it would not be possible for mothers to spend so long a time in hospital after delivery. This raised the question: if the mother goes home on the third or fourth day, will there be less breast-feeding? Might it be desirable to plan for new hospital and nursing procedures which encourage the mother immediately to assume the major care of her baby?

Thirdly, when members of the staff of the institution change, they pass through a period of uncertainty about their new service.

Another example of one-sided elaboration of practice is in the care of premature infants. Nowadays, the baby is removed quickly from the mother and completely taken care of by experts. Communication between mother and baby is cut off and the mother is faced with uncertainty about her future maternal role. Accepting the principles of increased maternal-baby communication will suggest a programme to be applied to institutional practices. For example the mother should be encouraged to send her milk to the baby, even though she cannot approach the baby herself. The nurse and doctor should give her a report once or twice a day while she is in hospital. It is important that she should see her baby at times, even through a glass panel. An early introduction to the visiting public health nurse should make for a clarification of their respective roles.

In the second year the child's task is mainly one of development, during which he learns self-respect, largely through his locomotor system, and through control of his involuntary muscle system. The problem here, in Erikson's phrase, is one of learned retention and release. When the child loses his sense of self-respect in this process, there results a sense of doubt and anxiety. At this stage of growth, parents customarily begin to exercise authority, often interpreted only as control, whereas the child himself seems to need the opportunity to make choices. When parents, or institutions, employ an authoritarian control, giving priority to their own needs, desires and goals, the child has less and less opportunity to make choices.

218

The need for continuity and time for this process of learning might be illustrated by an example: a child will stand in the middle of the hearthrug and urinate, in the presence of his mother, with an expression on his face suggesting that he knows what he is doing. His mother and those who support her have to learn that a child, in making choices, goes through three stages. In the first, he tells her after he has done the act. In the second, he tells her during the time he is doing it. In the final stages he will tell her before he does it.

This example can be applied to institutional practice among children between 1 and 4 years old, for the institution needs to have a sense of control. Hospitals have to control children in the sense of restricted activity, or immediate bathing, of holding for medication, and so on. Inevitably the implication of such control to the child might be expressed in the words, 'I am a thing'. Control should be modified to preserve a sense of autonomy in the child, a sense of 'I am William' and 'I am Mary' and 'they respect me and my feelings'. To prevent a loss of identity on his part the child must be aware that some of his needs, too, are being met by the control. Many children's hospitals, seeking to meet children's needs, have introduced play-rooms and play periods; in one, a nurse encouraged the young children to play with water and clay.

Institutions usually have a high sense of responsibility for the child and therefore their need to exercise control of the children is enhanced in a number of ways. In some ways institutions resemble minority groups and their specific needs must always be borne in mind when suggesting changes.

Many of the staff feelings, like those of minority groups, come from repressed tensions, and for example, can be shown by the staff of a mental deficiency institution in a number of different ways. A kind of martyr attitude is common: 'I have to give so much to the children in the institution' but underneath this is a feeling of lack of identification with the child. The staffs are liable to have a sense of isolation, which may well be carried across to the children themselves.

We cannot apply these principles to an institution without understanding the feelings of the staff. An order for a change of practice may be carried out to the letter, but if the staff have not been properly considered, the intention of the change may be lost. In a children's hospital we once proposed to change the visiting hours from once or twice a week to every day. The doctors in residence had discussed the matter together and some of them felt that the disturbance, unhappiness and emotional pain of the children when parents departed at visiting time was a reflection upon themselves. They had been particularly bothered when the child could not be comforted by their attentions, and they felt frustrated.

We asked the nurses whether they felt at times as if they themselves were the mothers of these children: a few replied that they thought of themselves as substitute mothers, but most of them admitted that they knew that they could not take the place of the mother. It finally emerged that both doctors and nurses had little desire to talk with the parents about their children. One nurse said, 'I get nervous talking about the children to their mothers', and another, 'I feel sorry when some mothers have to leave, and it makes me feel funny that I can stay here, even though it is my job.'·The resident doctor said, 'They ask me things that are non-medical.' These problems, which the staff have to face, need to be understood and the staff helped to bring them out and to clarify their attitude before a change is instituted; then they will work the new practice better. Where there is a conflict between the administrator and the nursing director of the ward, the staff finds it even more difficult to handle the painful feelings of children and parents.

The principles under discussion can have another application to the problems of staff adjustment and communication. One hospital which operates, for the health authority, a ward for crippled children, admits children of all ages from soon after birth up to 16 years, for periods of from a few weeks to several months, depending upon the nature of the illness. The ward was described as unhappy, and it was said that the parents seemed uneasy about their children. They felt that the attitude of the nurse in charge of the ward had something to do with it. We had a number of discussions with this nurse but there was no improvement. I visited the ward, found it very clean, very quiet, and the personnel were pleasant but guarded. The nurse-director of the ward was rather aloof and somewhat alarmed by my visit. I asked her how she felt about the ward and she admitted that she was worried. She had discussed the matter with the nurses without result. The parents were allowed to visit only once a week, and then for two hours. Some parents would stay outside the windows at other times to get a glimpse of their children.

We drew up a plan, with the co-operation of the Director of the hospital, the Director of the nurses, and the Director of the ward, to have a series of discussions led by experts corresponding to the professions of the members of the ward staff, but not associated with the hospital. The nurses were willing to give up free time. At the discussion certain principles were enunciated about the behaviour of the children and the talk centred round the examples of behaviour described by the staff. It became apparent to us that the punishments used were isolation and deprivation of privileges; the children had no group life except in so far as there were three or four in the same room. Any regression in toilet cleanliness was handled mainly by shaming and by the anger of the staff. Masturbation, especially among the girls, was said to be common. The nurses were in two camps, one identified with the superintendent and the other not, but unable to express their feelings about this.

At my next visit, five months later, I went in by a back way and the first thing I heard was the voices of the children in this ward. The voices indicated freedom of expression, laughter, and crying of an impatient quality. There were papers and toys on the floor and some litter around the beds, and a piano in the adjacent hall. The Director of the hospital said that after the discussions, things had gone along fairly well for two months and then destructive aggression in the children burst out again. This time he and the Director of Nurses, having taken part in the discussion groups, knew what the problem was and its chief source and were able to ask objectively for the resignation of the head nurse of the ward. As a result of the discussions, they had realized this nurse's limitation: they felt that the nurses themselves were really in sympathy with the Administration and wanted to change, provided the proper support were given.

After the resignation of the head nurse, the problem was solved and the atmosphere in the ward changed. The function of the discussion meeting had been to acquire information about the attitudes and practices of the staff which would need to be considered if any real change were to be made. Staff feelings of anger, resentment and fear of reprisal may be inhibited, but are transmitted surely and quickly to the children, just as such feelings of parents are communicated to their children. I believe that time must be taken and skilled methods introduced to clarify such staff feelings, if institutions are to help young children handle and accept their own feelings, already mobilized, of being ill or without their parents.

HEALTH EDUCATION IN CHILD WELFARE WORK

Including an Introduction to the Film 'Life Begins in Leeds' [1]

A. G. Joselin

MR. JOSELIN, in a brief description of the experiences of the makers of the film, said that ideas were gathered from the social field, the historical and geographical background, and the medical and psychological side respectively, by three sub-committees, and then made over to the photographer, Mr. Micklethwaite of the Yorkshire Film Company; Mrs. Mestel, of Leeds University, for contacts; and Mr. Joselin for direction.

It was not possible to write a proper script before starting shooting. Neither the exact locations for shooting, nor the kinds of sequences of activity which would be available were known. It was only possible to have in mind a draft theme, and then make contacts with the various authorities and homes, clinics and organizations.

Fortunately the photographer was one of those rare people who can go into a difficult situation and dissolve the tensions, and luckily the weather was remarkably good.

Wonderful co-operation was given by the local authority, the voluntary organizations, and private individuals. Some of the sequences were, in a way, private and confidential, and could only be obtained by assuring the mother or the group concerned that the film was for medical and psychological purposes and would not be shown in public.

DISCUSSION

All the contributors to the discussion congratulated the Leeds team on producing such a significant film with such meagre resources. It was calculated that the cost of the film, if made professionally, would have been not less than £6,000, whereas its actual cost was a little more than £300.

The film showed that one of the major social problems in Leeds is caused by the many houses still in use there which were built back-to-back some seventy-five years ago. Housing statistics show that these houses were condemned before the war, but owing to

[1] A technical documentary film specially prepared for the Seminar, and directed by A. G. Joselin. It shows various aspects of child welfare work in the City of Leeds. See Film List, p. 297.

222

post-war difficulties there are still more than 10,000 in occupation. It would have been interesting to have included in the film a shot of one of the small rooms in these houses, empty as when it was new. This would have given some idea of what the people coming from the country into the city seventy-five years ago would have faced, with their few possessions, when they began a new life in the town. By contrast, the shots of the rooms filled now with drawing-room suite, dining-room table, radio, washing machine, perambulator, and the many other gadgets of modern life considered to be necessities, would show how changes in living habits will create a problem which did not exist at the outset.

The first inhabitants of these houses were faced with problems over their children's health and food, but nowadays we know how to teach mothers and the mothers are willing to come and learn. The standard of child health is greatly improved and nutrition is no longer a problem. But the housing problem remains. The situation is all the more perplexing because the housing itself was not a problem originally, but it is now the hard core of all the social problems met with in this sphere.

Shots of this kind would have given a film more meaning to people from other parts of the world where there are also material difficulties, but different ones. The portrayal of the situation in Leeds would have been rounded off, moreover, by shots giving an impression of soot and rain and cold, to counteract the possibly false impression given by the continuous sunshine with which the film makers were blessed.

It was interesting to see in the film the young mothers in the antenatal and child welfare clinics, being taught about their pregnancy, and about baby care. It would be interesting to know what proportion of mothers do not attend such clinics, and whether those who do not attend might be just the ones whom one would like to influence most.

Little has been said about contact with the young fathers; perhaps the way of getting contact with everyone likely to make a home and have babies is in the top classes of the ordinary schools.

Swedish schools devote time to the subject called 'Family Knowledge', in which boys and girls of about 15 are taught how to make a family budget, how to plan a new home and buy furniture, how to take care of babies, and the need for a sense of responsibility for a family and children, and the importance of a good and affectionate spirit in the home.

Another question is whether the staff of the ante-natal and child welfare clinics should take part in the education in the schools; or would it be better for the school children merely to visit the clinics ?

It is probably true that the families which do not attend the clinics are those who most need the information and help, and in Leeds they may amount to 20 per cent of the whole. The most successful part of the educational programmes has been in regard to food.

Health visitors go to every family where a baby is born, and in addition, literature is sent by the Public Health Department to all families. In all types of schools there are classes for girls on the subjects of home-making, baby-rearing and so on.

In the U.K. other bodies such as the Marriage Guidance Council and Youth Clubs join in this educational work, and when the same people give instruction in the schools as in the clinics, this helps to give continuity. Unfortunately in Leeds in the boys' schools no instruction is given about the care of children, but only to some small extent, sex instruction.

In various cities in France, and in Algiers, schools for parents have been established, though it is doubtful whether the methods employed are very useful. It is, perhaps, more useful to organize small groups of parents to have brief lectures leading to a discussion. This allows each parent to explain and to relive his or her own personal experience and discuss it, not only with the lecturer but with the other parents present.

The salient problem in mental hygiene education is how to present information in a form that people can use. Experience of teaching medical students suggests that people cannot accept knowledge about mental health unless they have in some way experienced the situation under discussion; human powers of forgetting and suppressing are marvellous. If the students are in small groups, so that they can experience something of the emotions which come from a real discussion of those problems, the information may come to mean something to them.

There are other difficulties in the way. Cheap literature, magazines and films present to young people the idea that true love turns the world into a rose-tinted place, where happiness and security last until old age. When their marriage is not going well and they turn to their friends and parents for advice, they are frequently told that if they have a child all will be well. But what a preparation to have a child! Great strides have been made in preparing women and young girls for pregnancy, childbirth and child-rearing, but there are still very strong prejudices, folk-lore, fears and anxieties, to be contended with. Dr. Mead has remarked that instinct, even in the primitive tribes, has very little to do with child-rearing practices; that the mother knows very little instinctively, but relies on tradition. We tend to assume that it is unnecessary to teach mothers how to look after their babies, but this is not true.

Part Six

TECHNIQUES FOR CHANGING
SOCIAL PRACTICES

MENTAL HYGIENE IMPLICATIONS
OF POLICIES LEADING TO CHANGE
OF SOCIAL PRACTICES

Kent A. Zimmerman

IN CONSIDERING this subject I found that, logically, I could not proceed unless I considered first the mental hygiene implications of social change, so I will start by describing something of what has taken place in, and is concomitant with, the so-called mental hygiene movement in the United States.

The change of emphasis in mental hygiene might be said to fall into three phases, and each period has been characterized by one predominant interest. In the first phase, from 1900 to 1920, the emphasis was on improving the mental hospitals and on changing society's attitude of neglect and rejection of the mentally ill. The second period, 1920 to 1940, in addition, was the period of the child guidance clinic. Each community was urged to begin to plan for a clinic and, characteristically also, the role of the expert was generally over-emphasized. In the third, and present, phase of the mental hygiene movement, the emphasis has been on community mental health, and especially the family. Characteristic, too, is the theme that all professional workers in touch with families have as important and individual a role to play in family mental health as has the psychiatrist.

Moreover, I think that we do not contribute to our understanding of the development of a mental health movement in a culture, if we persist in thinking of it as an isolated movement. Such a movement is only one part of a wider and more comprehensive change. The behavioural sciences (of which psychiatry is but one) both influence, and are influenced by, such a change.

In the 1900 to 1920 period, psychiatry was mainly concerned with the nosological classification of mental disorders, and, at that time also, the legal aspect of psychiatric treatment was of almost predominant importance. Concepts of the primary causes of mental disease were almost entirely based upon pathological changes in body tissues. In many countries, children held a relatively inferior status, and were still exploited in industry, while their medical and

227

social care was poor. However, child labour laws and other social legislation for children began to change these conditions.

The years from 1920 to 1940 saw the impact on psychiatry of the dynamic theories of mental illness, especially as developed by the schools of Sigmund Freud and Adolph Meyer. These schools paid much attention to the nature of childhood experiences and their significance for adult health and illness. Furthermore, these dynamic theories led to the implication that other professional people, as well as psychiatrists, had very important contributions to make to mental health. Both Sigmund Freud and Adolph Meyer wrote excellent papers on the application of their concepts to education and the role of the school teacher. In these years, too, the nursery-school movement blossomed. An Italian physician, Dr. Maria Montessori, had a profound influence on nursery-school education and helped immensely to further the concept that the child is not a miniature adult but an individual in his own right.

In the present era, psychiatry has not only come out of its isolation from the other medical and social sciences, but has begun to offer itself for the service of professional people who, generally, do not have responsibility for the mentally ill: nurses, doctors, ministers of religion and priests, social workers, administrators, and the like. Social welfare programmes for children now stress the importance of family life, with the general theme that the child is but one member of the family, and his needs are best met when the needs of all the family are met.

I would emphasize that the mental hygiene movement and the changes which evolve in it are related to other contemporary cultural changes and scientific advances. Psychiatry and programmes for the social welfare of children both influence profoundly, and are in turn influenced by, mental hygiene programmes.

It is important to note that the programmes of the mental hygiene movement are not completed, and the goals not reached, in the phase in which the programmes begin. For example, although the care of the mentally ill in mental hospitals was the preoccupation between 1900 and 1920, no general improvement was attained in the U.S.A. until the years since 1940. Likewise, child guidance clinics, advocated in the period 1920–1940, are only in recent years being used wisely by the community. There remains a very real problem of consolidation of the older developments.

This leads us to the need for a balanced programme in mental hygiene, to the discovery that to over-emphasize one aspect of mental hygiene practice is to weaken the whole programme. Too much emphasis on providing mental hospitals or out-patient clinics will lead to the frustrating experience of finding that psychiatric treatment alone will never be sufficient. In the United States the goal for clinics that treat children has been one for every 100,000 and we now have one clinic per 110,000 to 115,000: but a recent U.S. Public Health Service report recommends a proportion of one per 50,000 people. On the other hand, too much emphasis on community education for earlier case finding and earlier acceptance of treatment results in people seeking resources that are not yet available. But since the provision of mental hospitals is not adequate for the needs of the community, we need to pay great attention to the role of non-psychiatric workers and of the general public, in mental health work.

In a complete programme the four sides of mental health work, hospitals, out-patient clinics, community education and education of the public, must not get out of proportion. We may well experience a sense of confusion when we assume responsibility for setting up mental health programmes. Anxiety may make us prone to rush into action with whatever seems reasonable at the moment; we may seize on one good idea to the exclusion of others. For example, some people believe that heredity is the major cause of mental illness and they advocate sterilization; others believe that we should increase the opportunity for religious experience in our communities. There are psychiatrists who say that the pressure of living must be reduced and that social planning is of vital importance. All these ideas are sound in many ways, but others are less sound. For example, people may advocate the abolition of most comic papers and certain kinds of television programmes; and to some it seems that as long as *something* is done, it is a mental hygiene programme.

Many people feel that the main emphasis in programmes should be given to children; but what should be emphasized? More breast-feeding; less separation from the mother; more permissive toilet-training; a father figure for every child? It is held that if enough is done for children, they will grow up mature adults and will themselves change social conditions; but anthropologists have shown that the community is not made up of the mere sum of its individuals but of interacting individuals. On this basis it seems reasonable not to devote all our attention to children but to help adults as well. However, when dealing with children, parents come into the picture and so the idea of parent education arises; but it might be as reasonable to put emphasis on grandparents, because many of the problems of parents stem from their incompletely worked-through relationships with their own parents. However, children have a longer life span and so may be more rewarding objects for our main attention.

Limited resources make a clear working concept of mental health a necessity. I have found it helpful to see in it three constituents:

first, the idea of the integration of the personality, that the internal adjustment of the person has been built up step by step, in an orderly progression, so that satisfying relationships are achieved with people important to him in his life; secondly, the existence of a dynamic force for mental health in each individual, which results in the individual's continued attempt to master his environment in all its aspects; thirdly, the need for the individual's relations with his cultural environment to be satisfactory.

Such a concept has relatively little emphasis on constitution or heredity, but it bears on relationships both within the family and in the community and also, beyond the family, in the institutions which serve the family.

In applying our working concept of mental health to the community, use can be made of what might be called 'psychological growth crises' in an individual's life. These crises come usually when the individual undergoes experiences which enrich or extend his personality, such as engagement, marriage, pregnancy, birth of a child; or the converse, experiences which impoverish or contract the personality, as in separation from a loved individual, bereavement and serious illness. Similarly in childhood there are certain normal learning experiences connected with growing independence from parents, such as weaning, toilet-training, the birth of a sibling and so forth. Adults and children undergoing these experiences, are in the process of further integration of their own life experience and are at these times highly educable, and are more responsive to people who approach them in such a capacity.

This notion, of increased capacity for learning and personality integration, can be joined with another concept, that in each community there are men and women who, by occupation and position are leaders or 'key people'. There are those who are in touch with people at these times of increased capacity for learning—physicians, nurses, ministers, school teachers, and so on; those who lead the institutions through which the professional people work—professional societies and social groups; and those who, though not officials, hold positions of influence in the community and form a 'network of influence'. The interest of these key persons in the mental hygiene programme has to be aroused, maintained, and kept in balance. How are we going to teach them or help them?

There are several ways of involving these key people. For example, by slogans; we can say: 'Keep all babies with their mothers until 3 years of age', 'Encourage fathers and mothers to love their children', 'Change as many mothers as possible from a rigid feeding schedule', 'Have a child guidance clinic for every 50,000 people', 'Use more foster mothers', and so on. But would the public health doctors, for example, appreciate being told these things? Moreover, there are certain dangers in slogans, in that the slogan itself may become the main point of interest to the administrator rather than the lesson behind it. Much effort may go to ensure that the slogan is carried out, and the slogan may come to be taken as being the whole programme of the organization. Thus, though the slogan may have been given by the psychiatrist, its meaning may have been imparted by the administrator.

Another danger about slogans is that they tend to increase standardization of approach. For instance, if we adopt the slogan 'change all mothers from rigid feeding schedules to self-demand', the implication is that of extremes, black or white, good or evil, and the real lesson is obscured. The slogan should be for the use of the individual, it should be put forward as a principle, with due regard to timing and the readiness of the people to use it. The slogan can easily become more important to the issuer than to the recipient, more associated with need of the former than of the latter, and used for the purposes of the former more often than of the latter.

The mental health movement itself brings pressures to bear upon people. It becomes our obligation to help people to cope with these pressures on themselves and not to develop more slogans and more pressures than people can stand. How do we manage this? The community mental health programme needs a basic principle of approach to allow it to be flexible in application to its many important aspects. This basic programme core is the parent-child relationship, our knowledge of which is now sufficient to give us something to work with. Our very way of imparting this knowledge will let people decide whether we mean what we say.

For real change to take place, people must be able to make their own choice. Kurt Lewin and his colleagues have shown that decisions made by a group tend to be identified by the individual with his own life goals more readily than decisions arrived at by lecture or other non-group methods. During the war, the U.S. government found it necessary for people to change their food habits radically. Dr. Lewin demonstrated that when group experience of change was offered, even those who all their life had eaten white bread, changed over to eating whole-wheat bread. This is our way of approach to the community through key persons. Moreover, people always have problems and in this there is an opportunity, because when people have problems and want help, they are highly receptive, highly educable, and willing to change.

What kind of problems can be found in the community groups enumerated? One problem of key people arises from community pressure. During the course of studying what mental health needs existed in California, I asked the health officers what they thought was needed, and discovered that they were being pressed by their communities for the rapid development of mental hygiene clinics and child guidance clinics. The health officers knew they could not provide either finance or personnel to the degree that the clinics needed. We proposed a meeting to discuss these problems. Twenty-two local health officers met with a team of psychiatrists. We spent two weeks together and then went our ways. Within two years, fifteen of the health officers had developed, or were participating in, mental health programmes in their communities, and in three years, eighteen had done so. Two had aided and abetted the starting of clinics; four added to their staffs part-time or full-time psychiatric consultants or psychiatric social workers, for use as consultants in case-problems and for helping to solve certain problems of inter-personal relationships; nine developed staff education programmes. As a result of this seminar, we had to develop group teaching techniques to use the shortest possible amount of time to provide a truly educational experience for staffs of public health depart-ments, an experience which would become an integral part of the person and would result in a change of attitude and change of work practice. We required participation by the group in planning our teaching programme, and we required two consecutive full days of staff time for our meetings. Our teaching of human relations was built up around the problems of relationships in their work, and our purpose was to define the alternatives between which they had to choose. In doing this, they furthered their understanding of patients' feelings by a better understanding of their own.

Another opportunity for useful educational work is in connection with the so called 'problem families' in the community, families in which the children suffer because their parents work out their own problems in the family. They are inadequate in their adjustment and contributions to the community, and they use up much of the community workers' energy and time. At St. Paul, Minnesota, it was found that a certain 6 per cent of the families in the community used 60 per cent of the time and services of the social agencies. Moreover, the problems of these families are usually not solved, and the worker remains with sufficient frustration to want to learn more about methods of work. Discussion about these problems can devolve around worker-agency-patient relationships and arrive at group decisions likely to contribute to the real professional growth of both supervisor and worker and, through them, to the life adjustment of the patient or client. This kind of education takes relatively longer to yield results, but is more permanent and more economical of staff time in the long run. One group took three years, meeting once a month for nine months in the year, to develop from the mere mechanics of supervision to the dynamic reasons for the behaviour of people.

To conclude: we are in a mental health movement at various stages of development and growth in different countries; all may not go through the same phases, but whatever phase we are in, we are certain to feel some confusion. If we resolve our confusion by applying the fundamental principles of our knowledge about personal and community mental health, we shall further the mental health, both of ourselves, and our fellow countrymen.

DISCUSSION

Developments such as have been described are difficult, if not impossible, in societies which are authoritarian throughout; but in partly authoritarian societies, the most effective way may be to work through groups of citizens independent of the government, groups without a vested interest in keeping things static. Mental hygiene societies, or parent/teacher organizations, or other groups of volunteers, often have within them persons who can bring pressure to bear and produce changes.

In pioneer work, the question should be asked: what are the most important characteristics of a mental health institution? The first essential is to discover the nature of the concepts of mental health, held among physicians, nurses, social workers, or interested citizens, and to relate the first steps to these concepts. These people might consider, for example, that the country needed more clinics, and in meeting that need, the opportunity might come to go further and to develop a non-clinical, so-called preventive, programme. The great principle is to start with what one already has and work along with that. It may be a handicap to apply too much the experience of highly industrialized countries to a country which is not ready for it. The important thing is to start strictly from the present position, to feel respect for the present and immediate past: each country and district is unique, and the problems of each must be solved in ways appropriate to each.

233

PANEL DISCUSSION ON EFFECTIVE
METHODS OF SECURING SOCIAL CHANGE

Leader: Kent A. Zimmerman

DR. ZIMMERMAN said that the members of the discussion panel came from five countries which were in various stages of development, and also from various professions and positions of leadership. Each panel member would give particular consideration to the social problems of his country, the concepts of mental hygiene there, and to his own opportunity to make a contribution to the development of mental hygiene.

DR. BARTHOLD HENGEVELD (*Netherlands*), paediatrician and public health officer: In his function of treating the child and advising the mother, the paediatrician should go beyond the symptom; but most paediatricians are untrained in dynamic psychology and look for help in this from psychiatric colleagues.

Even the change of medical attitude to the removal of tonsils and adenoids shows how great a change is taking place. Now it is held not only that a child should not have this operation before he is 6 years old, but it is also questioned whether the child should stay the night in hospital after the operation, or not be visited by his mother immediately after the operation. Many people have guilty feelings about the practice of taking children into hospital.

The whole community must take part in the enormous changes now going on; it is attitudes more than techniques which need to be changed; and the basic principles of dynamic psychology, expressed in common everyday language, must be kept in mind. But although attempts to influence paediatric colleagues may present greater difficulties than attempts to influence the parents, for the former do not all accept the evidence, such as that of the film *Grief*[1], they may well allow the treatment of the children under their care to be governed by more enlightened principles. The main opportunities in the Netherlands would be to influence the paediatric care of children.

DR. MARGUERITE CLAVEAU (*France*), public health doctor: The doctor in charge of a physical and mental health clinic, working on a limited budget, would find that the experience of the Seminar would give an orientation founded on fact and applicable to everyday

[1] See Film List, p. 297.

234

work. In a district in France, one social worker is responsible for mental welfare in an area containing 700,000 inhabitants, and her work must be limited to consultations in cases of mental disorder. But the general aim of the work is orientation in mental hygiene and re-establishment of the equilibrium of the families concerned.

The education of families is a vast, but highly interesting programme. In family clubs and parents' schools something can be done for the mental and general health of young children. We have assimilated modern knowledge of the difficulties and damage caused to children by separation from their mothers, and the social workers are trained to place children in families, when separation from their real families cannot be avoided. When building maternity wards, it is easy to arrange to keep the child's crib next to the mother, but it is not possible to replace overnight, institutions such as nurseries. However, the personnel can be trained to replace the present system on which they work with a system of substitute families, thus creating the necessary atmosphere for maintaining good mental hygiene.

DR. CHARIKLIA ALEXANDRAKI (*Greece*), Social Welfare Adviser to the Minister of Welfare: It is important for the adviser to take an active part in the work, otherwise it is not easy to work closely with administrators. There are many social changes taking place in Greece, as a result of the occupation and other great difficulties. During the war of 1940, the occupation, and the revolution in 1948, over 2,000 villages, that is more than 65 per cent of the houses, were destroyed, 175,000 refugees went from the country to the towns and there were 200,000 orphaned children. The first task has been to survive the emergency. The villages have had to be rebuilt and the people helped to repatriate themselves. The staff of government and voluntary organizations have become used to this exhausting emergency work, and have developed the kind of mentality which enjoys work that provides excitement and has to be finished quickly. In planning for long-term programmes this mental attitude has to be taken into consideration and the personnel given time to adjust themselves. Training courses are now planned to make clear that social work does not mean supplying people with the means to live, but rather helping them to become independent, to respect themselves and be respected. The family is the centre of the programme and public health nurses are given a certain amount of training regarding the family as a whole.

In Greece the term 'psychic health' is used rather than 'mental health', and this programme is thought of as preventive. The Ministry of Health and the Ministry of Welfare are co-ordinating their centres in the villages, to provide a visiting nurse and social workers.

My main task now will be with those administrators who separate in their minds the physical and psychological activities of a person's life.

DR. MOAMMER KHALID SHABENDER (*Iraq*), psychiatrist: Though Iraq has a long cultural history, it became an independent state only twenty-five years ago, after six centuries of domination by Mongols and Turks. The Iraqi Government had to build a new country from practically nothing. The public demanded improvement in every field of life, but at that time sanitation was unknown, and the community was illiterate except for a few officials educated so that they might run the local administration.

The land is exceedingly fertile, but only 5 per cent of the land was cultivated under the old regime and that in an old-fashioned way. By 1927 primary and secondary education had reached a good standard and in that year the first medical college was established. By 1952 there were 500 students in that college, one-fifth of whom were girls. About fifty doctors a year are now becoming qualified and some go abroad for higher qualifications. There is, as yet, no scheme for child guidance or for training social workers and psychiatric social workers, or for providing institutions for the mentally ill, but hospitals have been built and the standard of living in every direction has been raised. Now the necessity for establishing a scheme to promote mental hygiene is recognized.

As a psychiatrist working in a mental hospital, I take an active role in the Society of Child Welfare, I am editor of a journal intended to educate families in the physical and mental aspects of child welfare, and have prepared the way to establishing much needed child guidance clinics, institutions for mentally defective and other handicapped children, day-nurseries, and the training of social workers.

DR. PER ANCHERSON (*Norway*), psychiatrist and lecturer in social medicine: As a teacher I have become aware of the necessity of improving the quality of work in social medicine as well as extending legislation, but this latter would occur as a consequence of the work itself. My first task is to improve personal relationships in my own teaching hospital. During the last few years the general hospitals in Norway have become aware of the need for psychiatric services and it is significant that at a meeting in October, 1952, I read an introductory paper on the relationship between psychiatry and internal medicine in the hospitals.

It will be possible to influence public health policy so that the mental health education of the public health staff is improved, and the importance of the family recognized.

As special work, the successful attempt to introduce mental health principles, based on dynamic psychology, into sports associations can be mentioned. We have tried to canalize, in support of mental hygiene, the strong demand for physical activities in Norway, in terms of co-operation between the family, the school and the Church. The advantage of this in terms of a more mature adaptation to family life cannot be over-emphasized.

DR. ZIMMERMAN, in summing up, said that the panel had given a broader perspective of some of the problems to be faced in developing mental hygiene programmes.

DISCUSSION

In the course of the rapid evolution in Algeria, there is a danger there that medicine and hygiene may be regarded as instruments by which one civilization penetrates into another. Not all measures suitable for a highly developed people are applicable to a less highly developed people; for instance, it would be inopportune to establish child guidance clinics where the foundations of mental hygiene are still to be built. Innovations have to be made in such a way that the least possible resistance is aroused.

One of the aims of mental hygiene in such situations should be to create more independence of thought, to allow a local population to acquire more ease in their relationship with the governing classes, so that they could understand their own problems and deal with them.

The education of a country should begin from a nucleus in the country itself; European civilization can give advice and teach, but it should not impose its own ideas on other people. The soundest way to develop a people, a nation, a community, is to encourage them to develop through their own judgment and initiative.

The personality of those working in mental hygiene has to be considered: not only psychiatrists, but social workers, teachers, lawyers, and all those who might be regarded as key people. Something can be done by selecting administrators with suitable personalities, but key people already there cannot be trained because they are already in superior positions, although their personalities may be unsuitable for this kind of work. However, can it be said which kinds of personalities are most suitable to be entrusted with administrative power? It would be interesting to know which kind of people create the most difficulties; psychopathic personalities, people with insecure personalities, or those who are paranoid? Such people in positions of power can be a great danger to the mental hygiene of the country itself. It might be that neurotics, anxious and depressive people, are more dangerous to themselves than to other people, and perhaps the best administrators of mental hygiene are those who, though with some anxiety and depression, are in touch with reality.

SOCIAL WORK AND THE MENTAL HYGIENE OF CHILDREN

Helvi Boothe

THE ROOTS of social work as a profession reach deeply into the past. Some form of social work is to be found in all ages in which members of a society experienced disparity between their needs and their circumstances. In the twentieth century this profession has emerged from an unformulated, nebulous state and achieved a specific body of knowledge and specific tools, a conglomerate of many sciences, necessary to the essential purpose of helping people in need to mobilize their resources. These sciences have contributed to the formulation of the concept of 'case work', a social work tool which must be explained in relation to mental hygiene work with children.

The history of social work in Great Britain and the United States reveals that some form of case work has been used for a long time. As recently as the latter half of the nineteenth century, however, case work practice was still only a method of giving help to the indigent, and on this materialistic foundation is erected our present-day concept of case work. For two generations before the first World War, social work literature asserted from time to time that one may benefit permanently from assistance only if it ministers to one's psychological need. Pioneers of social work in still earlier days clearly realized their need to treat persons seeking help as individuals, and foresaw that knowledge would be acquired by which social workers might help their clients to effect better relations with other people and with their own environment. Unfortunately social work training for decades stubbornly resisted such progressive views.

American social workers are no longer an obscure group of 'do-gooders': they are to-day members of a publicly esteemed profession, with responsibilities, and with official recognition. A legislative framework for the new profession was erected during the depression years of the 1930's, and in the second World War the humane, scientific treatment of mental illness and personality disturbance in the armed forces greatly extended the professional relationship of the social workers and the psychiatrists. With all its new science and professionalism, social work needs the tempering influence of that humanitarian, ethical spirit which motivated its pioneers. Regard-

238

less of the new tools and the new circumstances, the essential social work responsibility is unchanged.

We are to examine social case work in its application to the problems of children. I shall consider the use of this instrument by the professionally trained social worker whose methods of contributing to the welfare of his clients are individual as well as social.

Perhaps the most familiar among all of the many definitions of case work is that given by Mary Richmond, in 1922: 'Social case work consists of those processes which develop personality through adjustment, consciously effected individual by individual, between men and their social environment.' This definition calls attention to one of the basic facts of case work, namely that it is not a profession in itself; it is a tool or a method developed for the purpose of discharging the obligations with which social work is charged. The case worker to-day engages to share in the process by which the client in need is to achieve a new equilibrium. Case work means to us a process of changing people in trouble; or rather, as Father Bower writes in the *Journal of Social Case Work* (November, 1949), 'the intrinsic end of its activity is a mobilization, an emancipation of the client's resources, enabling him to deal with his difficulties.' We know that without such mobilization of resources no material assistance can basically alter the client's situation or eliminate his trouble, and that to effect the change the social worker must understand the economic and social implications, and the laws and customs of the community to which his client belongs. He must also understand the dynamic force of his client's life experiences and the relationships between the client and the members of his family, his employer, his friends and his neighbours. A social worker, furthermore, must understand his own role and his own needs in his relations with his clients, and the effect of his own personality on the helping process. He is no longer handing out bits of material help or advice. He now participates, as Virginia Robinson says, 'in a reciprocal relationship in which he must accept himself and the other equally.'

It follows that to do his job the social worker must understand the forces both within and around the person in trouble. The social sciences play a predominant role in his basic equipment, he has also turned to psychiatry, not in order to employ new methods or to alter the basic purpose of the profession, but in order to develop necessary skills. Psychiatric concepts have become fused with the concept of case work to such a degree that to-day we cannot declare competent a case worker who does not understand personality development, and who does not possess at least some idea of deviations from the 'normal'.

239

Psychiatric social work is social work practised in direct working relation to psychiatry. Its content, method and purpose remain standard social work, but there is specific additional knowledge which the social worker needs to acquire when he collaborates with psychiatry. This is largely informational, including such subjects as the various syndromes of mental disease, psychiatric terminology, early symptomatology, psychiatric treatment methods. The psychiatric social worker needs to have more detailed information and understanding of the whole field of psychopathology than the social worker of other fields. All this is necessary in order that he may competently apply the basic professional skills acquired in his social work orientation and training, in the context of the psychiatric organization of which he is now a part. In a comparable manner adaptations of social work occur in other fields; for example the social worker in the school system or in the courts needs to acquire additional information equally accurate and specific.

I am deliberately stressing the importance of the broad common base of social case work and the relative unimportance of the additional knowledge required for the specific task. In the U.S.A. the young speciality of psychiatric social work has made a most significant contribution to the social work profession as a whole, but the psychiatric social worker has not always been an unmixed blessing because he has been confused about his identity and uncertain of his objectives. In the process of growth, psychiatric social work has faced the danger of losing contact with its mother profession as well as with its collaterals, such as nursing. To-day, far clearer about its origins and its objectives than fifteen years ago, psychiatric social work in the U.S.A. is ready, as an adaptation of the discipline of social work, to use its skills effectively in all appropriate fields of mental hygiene work.

The countries in which social work is still in a comparatively unformulated stage as a profession, might well benefit from this experience in the U.S.A., by careful differentiation between the basic body of knowledge necessary for all who engage in the process of helping people to change, and the detailed knowledge required by the specific agency. In other words, all social workers must have careful training in the skills of the 'helping process', in the understanding of human behaviour, including their own, and in normal and abnormal personality growth and change. It makes no difference to this requirement whether the adjustments and changes sought involve the environment alone, or also the internal structure and relationships of the people in need of help.

In describing what the social worker, thus trained, is equipped to do in his collaboration with child psychiatry, we frequently see references to 'social investigation'. 'History taking' seems to be one of the easiest social work jobs for non-social workers to comprehend, but this skill, too, has changed significantly. Whereas the histories of yesterday were mountains of data, to-day's histories are selective and dynamic accounts of the development of the person. Our knowledge of human behaviour has taught us that a 'fact' in the patient's life is a complex concept and not the absolute for which we used to take it. For example, once we might have recorded that Johnny's mother smacked him when he misbehaved, and gone on to great detail about the frequency and other characteristics of the punishment. To-day our interest would be not only in the details which surround the smacking but also in the mother's own feelings about them and in Johnny's reactions to the smacking. We know that the bare fact of smacking reveals very little about Johnny and his mother.

We say to-day that gathering relevant and accurate social information becomes possible when the informant's participation is obtained and when this participation is both conscious and spontaneous. Thus the trained social worker, fully accepting 'social investigation' as his job, nevertheless sees its chief importance in the specific context of informant participation and as the beginning phase of the relationship of receiving and giving help. What is the client's problem—not as we see it, but as he sees it, as he feels it? What does he want? Later, what is the agency prepared to do? Is it equipped to help the client, or will he be better served elsewhere?

A mother of a small boy comes to the child guidance clinic, referred by a teacher because of the boy's quarrelsome, aggressive behaviour in the schoolroom. To the social worker, who is the first one to see her in the clinic, she says belligerently, 'I came here because the teacher made the appointment and told me to come, but I want to tell you right now that it won't be any use. Jimmy is the spittin' image of his father and I can't do anything about it. They are both bullies.' The social worker obviously does not begin to gather 'social information', but sees that the mother, behind this belligerent front, is unhappy, bewildered and probably scared. He knows, furthermore, that any data secured from the mother at this point would be useless, because he would probably never lay eyes on the mother again. So he says instead: 'It must be annoying for a busy person like you to have to take the time to come here about something you feel may be hopeless. You have quite a problem, haven't you—two people bullying you? Or maybe it isn't a problem at all.' In some such a way he gets the mother talking; first, perhaps, just about how long it took her to get there, but as likely as not, fairly soon about herself, in more revealing ways. She eventually may even dare to say in her own words that she is lonely, unhappy and scared but that's just the way of things, and she does not know what to do about it. In fact, she is awfully worried because she knows that her husband once, in his 'teens, got into some trouble with the police, and now Jimmy seems to be going in the same direction. No matter how hard she smacks him, he simply won't stay in the house or play with nice boys in the park; he insists on tagging along with the big boys in the back alleys and bad streets.

She will go on about Jimmy's latest escapades, perhaps bragging about them while the social worker, watching his cues, may need to ask only a few directing questions or just register his interest. With a minimum of direct questioning, he obtains enough relevant information in a brief time to enable him to return to the original points: Does this mother see a problem in her family? Does she want to try to see if something can be done about it? Is this the appropriate place to help her to make the attempt? He tells the mother quite frankly that he also does not know whether she and Jimmy can be helped, but if she wants it, he would like to try. He gives her a simple explanation of the clinical services and then lets her make her own decision.

This preliminary process may take a long or a short time, depending on the particular characteristics of the mother and the skill of the interviewer. In any case, Jimmy's birth weight, eating habits or even the nature of his present problem is dead material until Jimmy's mother and Jimmy are actively and purposefully engaged in the effort to obtain help. In all phases of the helping process, the assistance is worthwhile only if it meets the existing needs of the person served. This fact obviously taxes the skill, sensitivity and ingenuity of the helping person, and often he fails in his effort. The failures perhaps even more than the successes reveal, by its conspicuous absence, the essential nature of this conscious personal involvement of the client.

To reiterate, in the context of the relationship established at the very start, the social worker receives the first necessary information which leads him to increasingly accurate insight into the forces operating. We no longer talk about this process as 'history taking' in a static sense, for the subtleties of the forces around the patient, and of his relationships within his family circle, neighbourhood and community, continue to be revealed throughout the therapeutic contact. In a way of speaking, our whole contact with the patient is a process of history taking: the entire contact of everyone in the clinic who works with the child and his family is dynamic and living, leading to ever-deepening understanding, while the therapeutic effect of having an interested and impartial listener begins at once.

An excellent illustration of this last point is the material furnished by the social worker in one of the French cases under study at the Seminar—Joelle D.[1] Here is a deeply troubled mother, not yet conscious of the effect of her own unhappiness on her child. Unfortunately the actual running account of the social worker's interviews is not available, and we cannot follow the social worker's technique step by step. The summarized results of the interviews reveal to us exceptionally rich material given by an unsophisticated mother who herself was astonished by her ability to speak frankly, because 'as a rule, she has great difficulty in making contacts with other people'. The visits 'stirred' her and 'brought something new into her solitary thought'.

Certainly here was a process far subtler than the gathering of data, a process which led this mother to ask for permission to keep in touch with the social worker about her problems with her child. Such a relationship is familiar to us from thousands of child guidance cases and we can foresee that this social worker is not going to offer this mother 'advice'. She is going to help her to continue talking about her problems as she feels them, to encourage her to discuss her wrong choices as well as her successes. In short, she will provide this lonely and desperate woman with an honest, trusting relationship with another human being who respects her rights of self-determination and her human dignity, and who does not reject her even when she does not measure up to some standard of behaviour she has set for herself. The experience does not solve Mrs. D's deep unconscious conflicts, but it may, nevertheless, bring about permanent changes in her feelings and subsequently in her behaviour towards those close to her.

The social worker here deals with conscious material, which the client brings into the interview, usually about the everyday environment. By confrontation, he may help the client to begin to see similarities between previously unthought-of situations in her own conscious reactions. He does not interpret the unconscious mechanisms behind the reactions, although his training must enable him to understand the client's personality make-up revealed in the conscious material, in order to be guided by it in his interviews. The social worker must be able to set the limits of the subject matter discussed, and at times skilfully guide the client away from potentially dangerous material which he is not equipped to handle.

The social worker is traditionally concerned with what our jargon calls 'the healthy part of the personality' which, after all, exists even in the sickest human being. He attempts to mobilize such strengths as the client has, in the hope of bringing about adjustment

[1] A case studied at the Seminar, but not included in Vol. II.

and change. He leaves it to the psychiatrist to change the course of the disease process itself, and concerns himself with the reactions of one member of the family on the other, and with the whole inter-reaction between the patient and his environment. We may recall that the social worker's collaboration with the psychiatrist arose from the observation of the psychiatrists in mental hospitals that some patients rapidly became worse after returning home as 'cured'. The importance of the forces within the family was revealed by this observation and social workers were engaged to attempt to help the family during the patient's hospitalization and after it, to meet and to solve the many problems related to the illness and the return of the patient to the community.

The concept that a child or an adult is not independent but a part of a whole—the family—is now familiar to all of us and it forms the framework within which the services of the social worker are given, whether he works with adults in a hospital clinic or with children and their parents in a child guidance centre.

I cannot attempt an exhaustive list of the ways in which the social worker is contributing to the work with children. Such services as selecting suitable foster homes for children and helping the foster parents in their period of adjustment to a strange child are common practice. In many places the social worker works with young mothers, individually as well as in groups, to help them gain confidence in their capacity to be good mothers.

However, it needs to be said explicitly that none of these processes should be considered the exclusive right of the social worker. In the U.S.A. there has been, in the last decade, much healthy inter-change of ideas and of techniques between the different disciplines engaged in helping people. Whether it is the social worker or the nurse, the health visitor or the almoner, the psychologist or the psychiatrist, who bears the responsibility of the helping process, is of secondary importance and may have to be decided—often on the basis of available personnel—by each country in its own way.

In conclusion, let me repeat and emphasize that there is an ever-growing conviction among the social workers in the U.S.A. that in order to bring about any lasting behaviour change such as an im-proved mother-child relationship, the help has to be given in the context of an understood and consciously directed relationship, in which the recipient is actively and willingly participating and which ministers to his psychological needs.

SELECTION AND TRAINING OF PROFESSIONAL WORKERS

Margaret Adams

THE PURPOSE of this brief paper is to identify for discussion some of the broad areas which might be of common interest and concern in the selection and training of professional workers.

In the U.S.A. we are constantly told over the radio and in the press that we need more psychiatrists, teachers, social workers, nurses, general practitioners, and the like. By comparison, there seems to be only a handful of people from our high schools, each year, to be recruited for these professions. It is possibly true of other countries too, that no profession can achieve its goal in relation to the number of workers.

This means that we must most critically examine our objectives for training, techniques of selection, length of training, methods of teaching, the concept of the role of the profession in society and of the relationship of the professions one to another.

Starting with recruitment we might ask whether we have adequate methods for determining the motivations which bring people to choose a particular profession? Is there an important self-selecting process, and what factors influence it? Can the professional groups interpret to the public what it means to be a member of the profession? Do we know how much the prospective student knows about the profession?

There is much dissatisfaction with current methods of professional selection. One School of Social Work has studied extensively the selection of students, and especially the method of personal interview. Each year former graduates of the school return for specialized training in interviewing techniques, with the aim of establishing throughout the country a network of these graduates. It might then be possible to arrange for a personal interview of a prospective student near his home, which would have great advantages for the individual as well as for the profession.

A professional school must recruit and select students in relation to some goal. A professional group should be able to formulate some concept of its role in society; but how? It has been said that professions must keep abreast of the changes within the social structure;

245

but each profession has the responsibility to interpret to society the role which it wishes to fulfil; to create an awareness of the need for services.

It is often held that each profession should be able to identify that which is its unique contribution to society; but can any profession do this alone? Is the main criterion that of services to people; and may we hope that to an ever-increasing degree, professional groups will together make these important decisions about commitment to services?

The relationship between professions often poses problems for both the professional workers and the recipients of the services. There are, for example, difficulties in the relationship between the nurse and the social worker. Often there is only one worker available, and this fact would largely determine the functions performed by the worker. This, however, might not be the basis upon which either nurses or social workers would choose to determine their respective roles.

Let us take an illustrative case of a child of school age who is in serious need of glasses, which he has not got in spite of the school's efforts to procure them. There are younger children in the family who have not yet been immunized. Unemployment and housing are also family problems.

One might wish to avoid having the family visited by too many different workers. Assuming a public health nurse and a social worker to be available, who should make the initial contact with the family? Would it not be possible for the nurse and social worker at the outset, together to set a tentative 'priority'? It might be decided that the nurse should make the first visit, it being understood that the nurse should work within the limits of her professional preparation. Subsequently, in conference with the social worker, they would plan the best way to aid the family and to support each other as professional workers. Thus, consultation rather than competition between public health nurse and social worker would ensure better service for the family.

Other questions arise in the relationships between any two professional groups. For example, does the problem of professional status tend to arise more frequently and with greater intensity between workers who are not well prepared? Does emotional maturity also influence the nature of the professional relationship?

I believe that if during training, nurses, doctors, social workers, teachers and others had more opportunity for joint discussions, a process of sharing and mutual understanding would result. This may be more difficult to achieve after qualification, when professional status may create difficulties in effective discussions. During training, however, they may be better able to focus upon the common problems without concern for professional status.

It sometimes becomes necessary to clarify 'role and function' within a given group. For example, in the nursing profession in the U.S.A. there are graduate and undergraduate professional nurses, less highly trained practical nurses, and other auxiliary workers. Bearing in mind the needs of the patient, it is not always as simple to allocate responsibilities within these groups as it might at first appear.

A patient's reaction to having an enema may necessitate the services of a nurse with awareness of some of the underlying causes of the patient's behaviour. A patient's defence against illness might result in 'withdrawal'. In the contact made with a patient during the giving of a bath or the making of a bed, a skilful nurse might get some cues as to the nature of the patient's anxiety. Yet on the basis of 'activities' alone, a practical nurse or auxiliary worker might have been considered sufficiently competent.

A student selects a 'profession', but in the professional training school he tests his previous image of what the profession is, what values it holds. The methods of teaching used and the relationships between students and faculty, therefore, are of tremendous significance. No learning takes place without self-involvement, and with rapid advances in knowledge, all professional people are confronted with problems in practice for which they were not prepared in training. Therefore, the development of problem-solving skills becomes increasingly important.

How close to reality can the professional training come? Some believe that through carefully planned and supervised 'field experience' students have an opportunity to discover for themselves what practice in a given profession is like; others believe this may be accomplished through seminars devoted to the discussion of 'real' situations; or some combination of these two methods may be advocated.

How the 'content' is evolved in a curriculum, how to evaluate the total curriculum, what is the responsibility of professional people 'in practice' to keep their respective schools informed of what actually happens, are all matters of concern to faculty members.

There is a widespread opinion that the professions should become more aware of responsibility for the personal development of students. More emphasis has been placed upon what society expects of these individuals than on their 'understanding' of the nature of their service. Might it not be that only those teachers who have experienced understanding can give understanding?

In teaching we place emphasis upon 'meeting the needs' of people. We recognize that no situation or behaviour may have the same meaning to any two people. This implies that if we are to meet individual needs we must always be asking 'what does an experience mean?' This idea might be illustrated by an experience in a paediatric ward, among children awaiting tonsillectomy. With each child's turn to go to the operating theatre, a staff nurse went to the bed to help the children and the student nurse who was caring for them. In one corner of the room Charles was sitting up in bed reading. Occasionally he looked around the ward. Soon, he put his book down and slid under the bed covers pulling the sheet over his head. The student nurse said, 'Charles is cold, I'll get him a blanket.' The staff nurse raised the question, 'could it have any other meaning?'

It was found that Charles had become increasingly anxious as he watched the other children being taken from the ward, and he closed his mind to anxiety by covering his head.

In relationships established during the training period, and through instruction, the student may find a setting in which he can learn the meaning of 'change'. From his experience he may question whether he can change others, or make it possible for them to change themselves, and may know from experience, what kind of emotional climate makes it possible to change. It may also be that from his personal experience he will know how much it sometimes 'costs' a person to change himself. If he has experienced this he may not be so frightened in the face of hostility and resistance, his own and that of others.

DISCUSSION

Many who have gone through the experience of 'change' realize that in the future, professional workers must have a different training and a different role.

It is suggested, for example, that future workers should combine the functions of nurse and social worker rather than perpetuate the present type of health visitor.

One proposal under consideration in Britain, is that the future medico-social worker should have three years' nursing training before nursing registration, followed by two years' training in social science before public health registration. Alternatively, the third year of general nursing training should be integrated with the first year of social science training, in order to preserve a four-year training.

An Institute of Research in Nursing has been established at Columbia University, New York City. It is hoped that a substantial contribution to nursing education can be made through the service of this Institute.

Part Seven

STUDIES IN PSYCHOLOGY AND NEUROLOGY, AND AIDS TO EDUCATION

THE SPACE, TIME, LANGUAGE AND INTELLECT OF THE YOUNG CHILD

G. P. Meredith

THE CHILD'S OUTER WORLD

WHAT SORTS of facts are relevant to the space, time, language and intellect of the child? They are so simple and obvious that at first sight they appear trivial. The child has a body which has a certain size and shape, and certain capacities for movement. He is held, by gravity, to the earth's surface, or to some artificial support such as floor, bed, chair or perambulator which stands on the earth's surface. At any given moment he is surrounded by material bodies such as bed-clothes, furniture, carpet, walls, doors, windows, or perhaps grass and trees, as well as human beings, dogs, cats, birds, insects, etc., and perhaps by flowers, and other plants, or by books, pictures, toys, kitchen utensils and so forth. These bodies are all extended in space and many of them are capable of movement. In any case the child must move in order to reach them. It is this fact which gives rise to the problem of spatial development in his mentality. Space is not a self-sufficient entity but one kind of abstraction from the series of events which constitute the development of the human being.

Another kind of abstraction is time. Beginning with a simple alternation of feeding and sleeping, the events of development unfold into ever more diversified happenings. Some of these recur with fairly rhythmic regularity. Day and night, meals, baths, and —according to family habit—a few more events such as father's return from work, all these are punctuations in the time-line and provide a first time-scale against which the more irregularly occurring episodes are placed and measured. This 'measurement' is rough and uncertain at first but becomes increasingly precise, especially when language enters the range of experience and introduces temporal terms such as 'after breakfast', 'bed-time', 'to-morrow', 'yesterday', 'soon' and the like. Time becomes increasingly articulated until in school and adult life in our mechanized western civilization all our actions are tyrannically tied to a framework of clocks, calendars, time-tables, diaries and appointments. This tyranny closes in on the

251

child all too soon, reinforced by the intrusion of rigidly scheduled radio and television programmes into the home, patterning our most intimate domestic life. Here, then, we have the problem of temporal development, i.e., the articulation of the child's mental time and of his temporal language so as to engage in the gears of his environment. Hamlet's inability to act on the ghost's bidding at the moment presented by the environment may be viewed as a dislocation of subjective time from objective time. Hamlet projected his neurosis outwards 'the time is out of joint—oh cursed spite, that ever I was born to set it right.' Do we recognize sufficiently the tyranny exerted by objective time on the developing mind striving to follow its own flow and rhythm? We must revert to this point presently.

Our third abstraction is language. Why do I call it an abstraction? Because language never occurs by itself. We single out the linguistic aspect of intercourse between persons. There are vocal operations, sound waves in the air and auditory mechanisms. Or there are writing, marks on paper, and reading. To the linguist, the phonetician, the scholar, these are perhaps sufficient. These things constitute language. But to the anthropologist and the psychologist language is part of a total pattern of behavioural interaction between persons. In this pattern is involved the social history of the group which evolved the language, a history which largely determines the meanings of the words. There are also the mental state, intention and attitude of the speaker; his bearing, his gestures; his relation to the hearer; the context of the situation which has stimulated the utterance, and the attitude and response of the hearer. All these could be analysed in multitudinous detail. All participate in the speech-occasion, or, *mutatis mutandis*, in the occasion of written communication. Thus linguistic development in the child is rich in emotion, intention, need, gesture, human relations, objective situations, in a word, *contextual completeness*. Actual words, at an early age, may be so imperfect as to be unrecognizable to a linguist yet perfectly understood *in their context* by the mother. But language, by its very nature, early begets a *consciousness of language*, a consciousness of far greater precision than the consciousness of gesture, facial expression, etc., which reach comparable control only in the professional actor. Language is used not only for talking about objects but also for talking about language itself, whereas gesture cannot discuss gesture, expression cannot discuss expression. Thus language soon emerges as a quasi-independent stream of development. And whilst it brings all the rich possibilities of social intercourse, this very fact makes it potentially another tyranny. For any slowness or defect of development imposes an obvious and tragic handicap on the child in relation to his more normal fellows.

We could spend a very long time discussing language and its importance in the development of the child. The only aspect I would stress at the moment is the view of language as a dynamic factor in the child's environment. He grows in an environment of significant and articulate sound. As the fish is enveloped by water the child is enveloped by language.

It will be appreciated that I am adopting a centripetal approach. I am asking: what are the various environmental factors converging on the child, the specifics of the 'reality principle' with which his thinly protected ego must come to terms or disintegrate? Only by answering this question can we begin to formulate the central problem to which his development must provide the solution. His intellect, of course, will play an increasing part in working out the solution but only as an uneasy leader of an army of other forces. Intellect enters our theme, however, by another route: it is one more factor in the environment. The child is surrounded by other human beings who, however unreasonable, do, nevertheless, exert intellect. The environment is not merely an aggregate of bodies: it is, as it were, a live chess-board in which self-determined moves of some degree of rationality are made. The child finds that part of his problem of living is a problem of *predicting*, and that whilst intuitive mechanics enables him to predict the movement of inanimate bodies, and intuitive biology foretells to some extent the behaviour of cats and dogs, he must perforce become an intuitive psychologist and logician to predict the actions of human beings. Thus intellect assumes the role of an environmental force to which adjustment is necessary.

There are many more features of the environment, but these four—space, time, language and intellect—have been given me as my universe of discourse and, indeed, they provide more than enough matter for discussion. I have so far displayed them as factors of the environment. I have now to show their modes of ingression into the inner world of the nascent mind. But first a few words concerning their *inter-relations* while still regarded as environmental factors.

Space assumes a quasi-independent existence only when time is ignored. It expresses certain features of the environment when the latter can be regarded as static. (But not all features, for there is one important feature, viz: *quality* of which I have said nothing.) Space is commonly associated with the notion of *extension*. It is more satisfactory to develop our concept of space from the notion of *discreteness*. The environment consists of a multiplicity of distinguishable parts or bodies. Each body is discrete, that is, it has a bounding surface. This surface defines its form and separates it from other bodies or from the intervening medium. The form is apprehended by seeing and handling, sensory-motor events which take time, and we see already that space cannot be divorced from time. The infant explores shapes with his fingers, his mouth and his eyes and builds up conceptions of form which are quite as much tactile and proprioceptive as visual. And thus a world of discrete objects segregates itself for him. As development proceeds these acquire names. These names provide the first *nouns* (or 'substantives') of his language. We may say then that one important division of language is determined by the spatial factor of the environment.

A second division of language, namely the verb, is derived from the temporal factor. The real environment is not static, it is a sequence of events. 'Time' is a way of referring to the fact that any two events either happen together or happen one after the other, with or without some overlap. But if the environment has already been segregated into distinct bodies these 'events' are seen as interactions between bodies. The mother pours the milk. The cup falls on the floor. The cat jumps on the chair. These are events seen as performances by bodies. And an early generalization takes place when *father* pours the milk, the *doll* falls on the floor or the *dog* jumps on the chair. *Performances* are conceptually separated from *performers* and the *verb* is born, expressing *actions* independently of particular *agents*.

The temporal factor and the spatial factor also bring other linguistic developments, viz: adverbs and prepositions such as *now, here, to-morrow, far away, after, behind, near, through*, etc. Mankind required many thousands of years of linguistic development to achieve the conceptual isolation of these relations from the flux of events. The words which express these abstractions are mastered by the individual child in the first three years of life. Objectively this can be attributed to the continuous interplay between the linguistic, the spatial and the temporal factors in his environment, i.e., the continual use of these spatial and temporal adverbs and prepositions by his parents in the spatial and temporal contexts to which they apply. But there is always something of a subjective miracle in the ability of a 3-year-old brain to perform these feats of complex apprehension and isolation, and correctly to use the appropriate adverb or preposition when the next analogous context occurs. It is important to appreciate what goes on here. Parents who try to over-simplify the process by indulging in baby-talk are depriving the child of the hard crusts of linguistic stimulus on which his intellectual teeth should be toughened. At the same time we must bear in mind that a distressingly large number of parents—even those who have had plenty of educational advantages—indulge in habitually slovenly speech not only as regards pronunciation but also as regards syntax. We may ask whether it is not possible to extend the revolution which has taken place in the dietetic and medical education of mothers, through the work of clinics and health visitors, into the linguistic field. If the mother could appreciate that she herself is the child's first language-teacher with a fundamental influence on all his subsequent schooling, might she not respond to *linguistic guidance* as she already responds to dietetic and clinical guidance? The possibility is worth investigating.

The other great word-generating factor in the environment is *quality*. The colours, sounds, shapes, tastes, smells, virtues, dangers and so on, which give the environment its experimental qualities produce the whole family of *adjectives*. Here again an act of isolation is required, for qualities never occur alone but always in attachment to bodies. However, the isolation, for example, of *green* from apple, leaf, grass, etc., is more easy and direct than the isolation of the spatial and temporal adverbs and prepositions already discussed, and presents no special difficulties so far as the more purely physical qualities are concerned. Qualities with an ethical implication, however, such as *good, naughty, careful*, etc., bring us right up against the concrete fact that language is an important component in the mechanism by which the adult imposes his own code of ethics, whether crude or refined, on the developing character of the child. For those adjectives are not purely descriptive, they express adult *evaluations*. Moreover *in use* they seldom express any lofty ethic consciously thought out in the quiet of the evening or in church, but the *operative ethic* of the adult's actual character as revealed in the particular situation. Thus the child learns not what the parent would like him to learn of ideal ethics but the ethics of the actual situation in which child and adult are involved. The meanings which the child comes to attach to ethical adjectives are the meanings implicit in their use in that situation. For that is the way all meanings are learnt in the early stages of linguistic development. Perhaps this is merely an elaborate way of saying that 'actions speak louder than words', but the point is that words gain their meanings from actions.

We see, then, that we have an environment of unfolding events in which the distinguishable factors of space, time, quality, language, intellect and character can be isolated in thought, though all conjoined in the fact. Many more factors would have to be included in a comprehensive study, but these are enough to suggest the complexity of the problem of adjustment which faces the developing human organism. What remains to be discussed, viz: how the child deals with the task, will be examined in the light of two considerations of fundamental significance. The first is that the child *is* an organism, with all that this implies, and not a mere bundle of cybernetic mechanisms. The second is that the environment is not altogether indifferent nor blindly hostile, though indifferent and hostile factors are present in plenty. It contains a large component of deliberate and mostly benevolent *contrivance*. The child is in a home, a family, a community, a state. He does not face his problem alone. The mother's care in the home, the clinical provisions in the health services and the educational services of state or private organization, all supplement and amplify the self-initiated achievements of the individual child.

THE CHILD'S INNER WORLD

In discussing the inner achievements of the child in mastering his environment we are faced with many difficulties. Every psychological term which we might be tempted to use is confused by a long history of controversy, e.g., *reaction, instinct, libido, unconscious, ego,* etc. I cannot hope to make statements which will be both worth stating and uncontroversial. But I do not consider it my function here to make dogmatic statements. Rather is it my task to promote the kind of questioning which may lead to fruitful thinking. But we must have some kind of framework within which to formulate our questions. I shall establish this framework about two concepts which I am going to call the *environmental challenge* and the *situational manœuvre*.

Let me explain these concepts by means of a simile. Imagine a naval vessel steaming through enemy-infested waters. It is dark but the captain has a radar-screen giving him information about his surroundings. He also has charts showing the permanent features of the area. His task is to get through the area safely, repelling any attacks which may develop, but not attacking without provocation. What appears on the radar-screen, considered in relation to his own position and speed, defines a *situation*. In so far as it calls for action on his part it constitutes a *challenge*. He must respond by an appropriate *manœuvre*. The appropriateness is relative not only to the nature of the challenge but also to his own position, his speed and direction, his weapons and his reserves of power. He takes the appropriate action. The situation is resolved. But now a new situation develops, another challenge. A further appropriate action is called for, appropriate to the new disposition of forces. He performs a second manœuvre. And so it goes on. The whole voyage is a journey through a *situational flux*. We may regard this picture as a dramatization of the child's temporal passage through his flux of environmental situations, with the necessary reservations attaching to all analogies. For charts he has a store of *memory-traces*. For radar-screen he has an *inner world* of multi-sensory experiences. For speed he has a certain momentum of behavioural processes. The environment is offering him a continual sequence of fluctuating challenges, not all necessarily dangerous in a biological sense but all disturbing the equilibrium of his *milieu interne*, and all, therefore, demanding appropriate manœuvres on his part.

The child's task is complicated by the circumstance that, unlike the captain who can distinguish perfectly between his charts, which are static, and his radar-screen which presents mobile images, he—the child—has an inner world in which active memory-traces and current sensory impressions blend into a composite dynamic view in which past and present are inextricably confused—rather as if the ship's monkey had seized the charts and was playing with them inside the radar apparatus. It is worse than this, for many of the charts are artistic works of fabrication, not scientific works of cartography.

One important aspect of this analogy is that it brings out the point that the child does not adjust his behaviour in relation to the outer world but in relation to his inner world. The captain responds to the images on the radar-screen, not directly to the enemy ships. This point was brought out by Koffka[1] in his account of 'the behavioural environment'. But I think Koffka was inadequate in his account of 'the geographical environment'. If we are going to use the word 'environment' to refer to the totality of physical and geographical facts the word becomes too wide to have any precise use. Further, it is confusing to speak of the 'behavioural environment' when referring to something which is essentially a psycho-neural pattern *within* the organism. The mental and the material become hopelessly mixed. The word 'environment' is sufficiently useful to be worth an effort at clarification. Out of the totality of physical facts surrounding the organism there is a certain selection which is potentially *relevant* to the organism. Everything outside this selection may be described as 'below the threshold of relevance'. By 'relevance' I mean *capacity for evoking behavioural responses*. For example, cosmic rays are part of the physical surroundings but they are not part of the 'environment' in the foregoing sense except in the case of a physicist who has instruments for detecting them. Any effect they have on the organism is a bio-physical effect which he cannot avoid and to which he cannot respond. Thus the *environment*, whilst objective in content, is delimited in scope by the needs and capacities of the organism. This is different from Koffka's 'behavioural environment'. And I think it is nearer to the popular use of the term 'environment'.

See (27) in Bibliography, p. 299.

Thus for any given organism we have:

(i) the *totality of objective facts*, some relevant, most irrelevant;

(ii) the *environment*, i.e., the selection of relevant facts;

(iii) the *inner world*, which includes the introjection of the environment by perceptual processes but much more besides. The introjection is not on to an 'empty screen'. The screen is already patterned by memory and fantasy.

This 'inner world' may be regarded as the modern conceptual successor to the 'stream of consciousness' of William James. To-day we are more impressed by the role of the unconscious. And we have more precise axes of description on which to plot the contours of the inner world.

Occupying an apparently intermediate position between the environment and the inner world is the child's own body. This provides the sensory instruments by which the outer world is known and the motor apparatus by which manœuvres are performed. But in addition it makes three other contributions to the life of the inner world. First, a good deal of the surface of the body is directly visible to its owner and all of it is within range of manual contact. Second, the *interoceptors*, i.e., the internal sense-organs by which the processes in all the internal organs report themselves to the autonomic and central nervous systems, give a general *tone* to the inner world, a tone which may be mellow or harsh, calm or restless, exuberant or painful; a tone which saturates everything on the screen whether objective or subjective in origin. We all know what it is to take a 'jaundiced' view of things or to look at life through 'rose-coloured spectacles'. Third, the *proprioceptors* by which the muscles, tendons, joints and semi-circular canals report to the brain on their own actions and on the spatial orientation of the body, are of particular importance in relation to the *space of the inner world* and I shall revert to them later, for they concern the detailed structure of this space. The broader features are provided by the relation of the environmental perspective to the body-surface. The latter provides a more or less constant spatial framework bearing a peculiarly intimate relation to the ego. This framework serves as the focus for the *perspective of the spatial environment*. The introjections of the body-surface, and of the environment, on to the screen of the inner world are related in a way which lays the foundation of an *inner space*. With respect to inner space it is helpful to think of space in terms of the cartographer who divides up space into lines of latitude and longitude. For him space is not empty, it is something criss-crossed with lines and it is that concept I would like you to keep in mind in what follows. This inner space has very different properties from those of the environmental space, which in turn are different from those of total physical space. This latter difference is a mathematical one which does not concern us here. What concerns us is the introjection of the perspective space of the environment on to the screen of the inner world. We could learn a good deal about this from the symbolic use of space by artists. In so far as the artist uses perspective he is merely portraying the environment. But when he resorts to vertical lines to suggest aspiration or resurgence, horizontals to suggest quiescence and peace, and diagonals to suggest action or downfall, as well as in his use of curves, grouping and other spatial devices, he is tacitly relying not on objective space but on the space of the inner world. This space cannot be described in mathematical terms alone. True, it *has* an objective determinant, viz: the perspective of the environment. There are also two other objective determinants. First, *gravity* which, when transferred to the inner space by means of its effects on experience (the effects of falling, and the effort needed to climb against gravity) gives the inner space a *vertical polarization*. The up-and-down direction is different from all others. And second, *light* which is almost always brighter in the upper half of the field of view than in the lower half. This reinforces the vertical polarization due to gravity, but I am not aware of any researches into its specific effects. Add to these a more subjective determinant, the relative positions of the various portions of the human anatomy—the feet (which get dirty) at the base; the genital and excretory organs, sources of desire and shame; the stomach and heart, where emotions appear subjectively to be located; and, at the top, the calm controlling cerebrum. Anatomy reinforces the vertical polarization due to the physical determinants, by an emotive and almost ethical component. This has a marked effect on language. We speak of *base* motives and *lofty* ideals. We *sink* into iniquity or our spirits *rise*. If by some means we could conduct research into the inner space of the ancient Greeks and the ancient Hebrews I would hazard a guess that the space of the latter would be found to be intensely polarized in the *vertical* direction, whilst the Greeks would show much greater freedom of *lateral* mental movement. The reasons for this guess will be obvious in the religion and science of the two races.

Modern physics has accustomed us to the thought that space is not the empty featureless void of Newtonian doctrine. It is structured by gravitational gradients and electromagnetic forces and waves. We have some precedent, then, for formulating a conception of a *structured inner space*. Indeed the neural basis of psychological states would of itself compel us to locate these states in a highly structured space. I have tried to show that the *location* of the body in the environment, the *anatomy* of the body itself and the *receptor connections* of the surface, the viscera and the motor organs with the cortex, between them provide certain guides to the gross structure of the inner space. Clues to the detailed structure—and here we come nearer to our central subject, the child, of whom we might appear to have lost sight—are to be found in *physical movement* and in *social behaviour*. We have learnt from the experiences of congenitally blind persons whose sight has been operatively restored, that the *visual* perception of shape is not the instantaneous process which normal adults suppose. It takes months of painful learning. We are safe in assuming that the infant builds up his capacity for perceiving the spatial forms of objects by a slow process of correlations between visual and tactile impressions and proprioceptive sensations from the eye muscles, the hands, the tongue and the lips. As he starts to crawl, to walk, to run and to climb, he builds up the larger space of distance, direction and elevation, and comes to translate the visually foreshortened perspective space of his environment into the Euclidean space of bodily movement. Thus *movement* must be regarded as a principal generator of the inner space. I would suggest that precision in the structure of the inner space is one of the firmest foundations for adult rationality. I cannot prove this hypothesis nor can I elaborate it here, but if it may be adopted as a working assumption it points to two practical consequences:

(i) the need for encouraging all the movement of which the infant is capable, within the limits of safety,

(ii) the need for associating linguistic development with the child's movements.

The first of these recommendations speaks for itself and is justified on many grounds. The second needs a little explanation. Rignano has suggested that thinking may be regarded as *inner experimentation*. I would describe thinking more generally as the *introjection of bodily actions*. In the process of introjection language plays a crucial role. It enables actions to be given symbolical representation in the inner world, thus setting them free from the limitations of specific imagery. In so far as the child is helped by his parents to associate his own movements with precise verbs, adverbs and prepositions, the introjections of these movements become precise *mental operations*.

Bodily actions include not only the whole range of locomotor actions of limbs and trunk but also the extremely varied actions of the hands, in manipulating all that the environment offers—materials hard and soft, plastic and elastic, greasy and sticky, clean and dirty, inanimate, living and human, powders and liquids, froths and jellies, winds and flames, in all manner of inter-relations and inter-actions—the fitting of lids on saucepans, of buttons into button-holes, the turning of handles and the pressing of switches, the folding of paper, the breaking of sticks, the rolling of cloth, the pouring of liquids—one could continue the list indefinitely. The quantity of self-pedagogy in which the child indulges in the early years is prodigious. He establishes all the experiential foundations of physics, chemistry, biology, sociology and mathematics. The problems of the parent are obvious—the dangers and accidents and wastage do not allow these problems to be ignored. But it is also important that the *opportunities* should not be ignored. I would say that the artificial environment of glossy toys, which parents and relatives like to provide, means considerably less to the child than the opportunity to explore pots, pans, cupboards, taps, grass, trees, worms, frogs and all the other resources of the real environment. He is hungry for the knowledge of the properties of matter. And thus he develops a labyrinth of fine structure in his inner space.

I have left the impact of social behaviour to the last because it is so fully dealt with by others. To relate this impact to the development of the inner space, we might adapt the topological concepts of Kurt Lewin, but his use of the term 'space' is more metaphorical than mine. I should prefer to treat the development by extending the proprioceptive function. The proprioceptors report to the cerebrum on the pattern of every action performed by the body, from the grossest locomotion to the finest wink of the eye. Thus they cover the inner space with an exquisitely fine and intricate pattern of recorded movements, the basis of all our skills. Now in addition to all these muscular movements we have all manner of *mental operations* ceaselessly at work. There is a puzzle here which I have nowhere seen adequately discussed. I refer to the fact that *we can remember our own mental operations*. Ordinary memory of objective perceptions and external behaviour is not much of a puzzle: we assume that the impulses from the exteroceptors and proprioceptors leave permanent traces in the nervous system. But how does the brain receive and retain the impressions of its own operations? This is such a special phenomenon that I have coined a special name for it. The impression made by a mental operation I call an *Entypism*. Whatever its explanation it is an important fact. Now we operate mentally on certain *operanda* and produce new mental *constructs*. For example the elder of two children sees the baby receiving favours of which he himself is deprived. These impressions are his *operanda*. By a rapid mental operation he evolves a pattern of action: 'I will act like a baby'. This pattern is a *construct*. The whole process is

261

likely to be full of tension. The fact that the reaction is largely unconscious does not affect the issue. We are very little aware of most of our proprioceptive impressions. A *movement of introjected mental contents* has occurred: a constructive operation has been performed and this will leave its own *entypism*. Every such entypism will contribute its quota of fine structure to the inner space. Those which are emotionally charged, like the example given, will leave structures which are, so to speak, deeply engraved. A mind with many conflicts will have an inner space like a battle-ground furrowed with trenches and pitted with shell-holes. The inner space has to accommodate the structure of all the Freudian complexes and much else besides. It is the log-book of the captain's journey through the situational flux.

I have used the term 'social behaviour' to cover the whole field of personal interactions, including the earliest mother-child relation, and have tried to show that we cannot afford to treat the supposedly cognitive realm of intellectual experiences, the learning of objects, space, time and language, as separate from the orectic realm of inter- and intra-personal tension, conflict and enjoyment. It is only in language, and in analytical thought, that these aspects of mental life become separated. There may be some neuro-anatomical separation in the respective functions of the cortex and the thalamus, but since these areas perform in continuous inter-action, the psycho-neural *inner world* is always a blend of the two and its space is structured by both.

I have not attempted to treat these factors of space, time, language and intellect in a conventional or orthodox manner, nor shown how the child's *concepts* of space and time mature, how his language develops nor how his intellectual capacity is determined. I have tried to stress the *inter-action* of these four factors. One of them in particular, namely *language*, is an extremely variable social factor which markedly affects the development of the other three, and is completely subject to the linguistic capacities and habits and *policies* of the human environment. To me the recording of norms of achievement of children in these four factors is of less interest than the study of the means by which parents and teachers can, by deliberate policy, maximize the environmental opportunity and stimulation by which the growth of the child's inner world can be made rich and satisfying. If the child is to manœuvre his way through the situational flux with zest and courage, the early environmental challenge is of supreme importance. Let us see that his ship is well-equipped and that his apparatus is in good working-order. But let us also ensure that the waters provide plenty of challenges to keep him alert and moving.

262

DISCUSSION

Professor MacCalman said he could not let one point made by Professor Meredith pass unchallenged. Professor Meredith spoke about the dynamic view in which the past and present were inextricably fused, rather as if the ship's monkey had seized the charts and was playing with them inside the radar apparatus. The longer one examined the inner processes of human minds the more respect one had for the accuracy and ordered speed and appropriateness of the actions of the inner mind. Before the discoveries of science, automatic forces had seemed to be very much confused, but the more one learned about those forces of nature, the more the feeling of confusion was replaced by recognition of the ordered skill of nature itself, and the inevitability of these actions. The unconscious world that Freud discovered had its own scientific laws, and these were as accurate and precise as anything known in nature; they had only seemed confused to us because we knew so little about them.

THE NEURO-MUSCULAR DEVELOPMENT OF THE CHILD[1]

Cyrille Koupernik

I WISH TO START from the standpoint that the two factors of heredity and environment are not mutually exclusive and that both influence the development of the child. There is in the developing child some internal force, of the same nature as that which gives the foetus a working system of circulation and a breathing system ready to function immediately after birth. Actually, these systems go on developing after birth, and their elaboration and development are parallel to the phenomenon of development of the nervous system. The fact that this is a process of maturation explains in great part the consistency of the development, it is a constantly moving scale which leads us from the newly-born to the older child.

In the new-born child, there is a striking contrast between the perfection of the functions serving its own life and the imperfection of its relations with the outside world. On the one hand, its blood circulates the oxygen efficiently and feeds it, thanks to its circulatory system; on the other hand, the child's spontaneous motility is global, archaic and explosive; but within this unco-ordinated motility one group of functions develops immediately, i.e., those necessary for the alimentary functions. This, perhaps, is why Freud foresaw with luminous vision the importance of the oral stage; and why the first effective social gesture of the child will be its smile. In addition to this spontaneous motility at birth, there is some reflex activity, of which three examples are the startle reflex of Moro; the stepping reflex which has been studied in the U.S. by MacGraw and in France by André Thomas; and the grasp reflex of the closing of the hand.

Towards the end of the second year, the child has five of those essential attributes which differentiate man from animals:

1. He walks on his hind legs, a privilege which he shares with his distant relation, the monkey.

2. The fact that he walks on his hind legs allows him to use his 'fore-paws' as tools, on which fact our civilization is largely based;

[1] The lecture was illustrated by films on child development produced by Professor Illingworth (Sheffield).

cerebral localization around the motor area shows that the area of hand innervation is far more extensive than the size of the hand would suggest. Comparatively speaking, it is the most extensive part of the sensory motor system.

3. He can use a system of symbols in his social relationships, i.e., language.

4. He is capable of interpreting another system of symbols, that of images; he can correlate two dimensional pictures with their three dimensional originals.

5. The most important attribute is, that the child has a concept of what is I, and what is not I.

The history of evolution along this developmental path is that of an emergence from the archaic reflex of the new-born child to an act adapted to a function, i.e., from a sub-cortical to a cortical activity. It is the function of the cerebral cortex to co-ordinate what is useful to a function, and to inhibit and suppress what is useless or antagonistic. All voluntary movement is a matter of co-ordination of antagonistic muscles, e.g., in the grasping of an object by the hand, the flexion of the fingers is reduced and controlled by synergic contractions of the muscles extending the fingers and also by the muscles extending the wrist: an example of a co-ordinated functional movement.

The great Canadian neuro-surgeon, Wilder Penfield, while operating on epileptics, found that the stimulation of a particular point on the temporal lobe brought about in the patients an experience from the past or a hallucination which was close to a dream state. This is a fascinating example of a connection between the constitution and an environmental experience. Constitution has determined the place of the temporal lobe in the phenomenon of memory, but the extent of the memory is brought about by the experience of the individual.

If our attitude to these matters is solely concerned with what the child *does*, we risk attaching equal importance to phenomena which have widely different values; which is the danger of too psychometric an attitude. Constitution must be considered together with environmental experience in establishing the norms of development, such as those which Arnold Gesell has formulated, to our lasting gratitude. Constitutional factors are fairly constant from one patient to another, within the different spheres of development: both in the sequence of development and in the way in which phenomena appear consecutively.

Variations of the environment have to be considerable before they can affect the development of a very young child. The biologically determined sequence is constant from one child to another, but the rhythm of development varies and thus the first sign of individuality appears. Moreover each family environment constitutes a unique psychological constellation and this provides us with the second environmental component of personality. No human being can be compared exactly with another.

There may also be pathological deviations to be considered, those of children whose brains have been damaged congenitally, in intrauterine life, during, or after birth; and the deviations of children whose environment has been so poor, or so abnormal, that their scale of development has been distorted.

In the neurological examination of a child we use two types of techniques: a fairly passive study of his muscle tone, and tests in which we can see how he functions within a standardized situation.

The common techniques of neurological examination may be outlined briefly in two groups, arranged in the sequence of developing function.

First:

1. General motility.
2. Muscle tone.
3. Posture.
4. Deep reflexes; plantar reflexes.
5. Archaic reflexes.
    (a) Moro or startle-reflex.
    (b) Stepping reflex.
    (c) Grasping reflex.

The deep reflexes and plantar reflexes are not much use in the examination of a very young child, for they are nearly always lively and diffuse. With regard to the startle reflex, also known as the embrace reflex, a child will respond in the same way to very different stimuli, spreading out its arms simultaneously and bringing them together again. This response is also bound up with a modification in the position of the head as has been illustrated by André Thomas; but that might also be regarded as a response to an auditory stimulus.

Next:

6. Prehension and manipulation.
7. Oculo-motor development.
8. Facial mimicry.
9. Play and use of tools.
10. Pictures.
11. Identification with the adult.

266

The inclusion of play and use of tools draws attention to the fact that we should not limit our examination to the reflexes.

Muscle tone can be gauged by the angle which can be formed between the thighs, which, in the baby, is not more than 40 degrees, and in a young child, never more than 90 degrees; whereas in the period of physiological hypotonus at the end of the second year, the child can not only do the splits but can put its foot on its shoulder. This is an indication of the postural or motor age of the child.

In the young infant, the muscular tone of the back is hypotonic and because of hypertonus of the flexors of the lower limbs, he cannot stretch them when sitting. Later on, the back becomes straighter and the child can stretch out the lower limbs.

There are three interesting ways of measuring the level of postural development of the child. First, in the first 2 months of life there is a generally noticeable asymmetry, the child's head being turned towards one side. Later on, at 4 months he becomes symmetrical and, finally, can move both ways independently. Secondly, if one pulls a young child to a sitting position, the head will fall backwards. At 5 months, he can maintain his head in line with his back. Thirdly, 'the dive': while holding the trunk, if the child's head is dropped towards the ground, without touching the ground, a child of 10 months will respond by spreading the arms.

However, there are no narrowly defined norms for development. For instance, some children will walk at 9 months, others at 18 months, but the child who does not walk until 18 months is not abnormal.

In the new-born child there is a certain sensitivity to light: in the presence of a bright light the new-born child will look at it fixedly and then go back to an intermediate position. At the age of 3 months the control of the oculo-motor muscles is quite organized and the eye of the child can sweep the whole horizon. In the new-born child only the muscles of the mouth have any co-ordinated motion, the rest is purely reflex. The first social smile appears between 1 and 2 months old; and around the age of 1 year, voluntary mimicry is seen—the child wants to clown and to imitate some of the expressions of the adult.

There are three development sequences of value in examination:

I. The reactions of the child to the human face:

   (i) Social smile at under 2 months.

   (ii) He will pat his mother's face at 3 months.

   (iii) Smile at his own face in the mirror at about 4 months.

   (iv) At 18 or 20 months he will recognize himself in a mirror.

(v) Towards the end of the second year he will recognize his own picture and that of people he knows.

II. The sequence of evolution from simple motor movements to elaborate gestures:

    (i) Play with the hands.

    (ii) Taking an object.

    (iii) Play, with an organized sequence of events.

    (iv) Throwing.

    (v) Paper-tearing.

    (vi) Putting a cube in a cup (end of the first year).

    (vii) Analysis of an object by the hand or finger.

    (viii) Rational use of tools (middle of the second year).

    (ix) Recognizes a teddy bear or a doll.

    (x) Dramatic play, playing at feeding the dolls or animals.

    (xi) An interest in pictures.

    (xii) An attempt at identification with the adult, e.g., when the young child pretends to read a newspaper by putting it in front of his eyes.

III. The development of language.

    (i) Babbling noises.

    (ii) Syllabic sounds.

    (iii) Jargon by which he learns to speak.

    (iv) Using two words together.

    (v) Three-word sentences.

    (vi) He calls himself by his first name.

    (vii) 'I' and 'you' pronouns.

THE DEVELOPMENT OF THE CHILD

A Pro-forma of Examination, by Cyrille Koupernik

I. NEUROLOGICAL EXAMINATION OF THE NEWBORN BABY

(1) General activity   (restless—normal—inactive)
    Sleep
    Crying   (exaggerated—weak)
    Pulse
    Respiration
    Temperature

Curve of growth, by weight
Cyanosis
Jaundice

(2) Movements   (slow—unco-ordinated—sharp)
    Abnormal movements   (fits—spasms of hypertonus)
    Muscle tone   (hypertonic—hypotonic)
       Head   (balanced—asymmetrical)
       Trunk
       Limbs
    Archaic reflexes
       Walking
       Stretching
       Startle (Moro)
       Grasping

II. EXAMINATION TECHNIQUES

(1) *Interview with mother*

    Somatic factors—Pregnancy
                    Confinement
                    State of baby at birth
                    First days of life
                    Development—to present day
                    Heredity—neurological diseases,
                                      malformations
    Social and Psychological factors (ad lib)

(2) *Examination of the baby*

    (a) *Neurological Examination*

        General activity
        Muscle tone
        Posture and movements
        Deep reflexes
        Skin reflexes
        Archaic reflexes
        Prehension
        Eye movements
        Facial mimicry
        Vegetative nervous system
            Temperature
            Sweating
            Dribbling

(b) *Psychological Examination*

Attitude towards tester
Attitude towards mother
Attitude towards test material
Attitude towards the neurological examination
Type of play—motor
                         combination of objects together
                         use of tools
                         animistic (make-believe)
                         reaction to pictures
                         reaction to mirror
                         reaction to photographs
Language

III. DETAILED NEUROLOGICAL EXAMINATION

(1) *Posture and locomotion*

Supine
Prone
Suspended in prone position
Pull to sit
Sitting
Standing
Walking with help
Walking alone (running and climbing stairs)
Diving reflex

(2) *Prehension (grasping)*

	Approximate normal age (in months)
Clenches fists	2—
Moves arms when sees an object	3
Two-handed grasping	4 ⌐
One-handed grasping	6
Cubito-palmar (ulnar)	4–5
Palmar	6
Radio-palmar	7–8
Radio-digital (thumb-forefinger)	8–9
An object in each hand	6
Transfer from hand to hand	6
Voluntary release of object	10+
Throwing objects	11+
Exploration by finger	10+

(3) *Oculo-motor development*

Phototropic nystagmus	Newborn
Oculo-motor control (fixation)	3

(4) *Facial Movements*

Muscles of the mouth and eyelids	Newborn
First socially adapted facial expression	1–2
Voluntary facial mimicry— imitation	11+

(5) *Reaction to auditory stimuli*

Mass reaction	Newborn
Facial reaction	2
Turns head and eyes towards stimulus	5–6

(6) *Reaction to human face*

First social smile	1–2
Smile at own face in mirror	4
Pats his picture	6
Identifies familiar faces in mirror	12–15 (?)
Identifies himself in mirror	18–24
Identifies familiar faces in photograph	18–21
Identifies himself in a photograph	20–24

(7) *Play*

Play with hands	3
Banging	6–7
Sequence of play	10
Throwing objects	11
Tears paper	10
Puts cube in cup	10–11
Puts pellet in bottle	15
Takes pellet out of bottle	18
Examines objects by finger	10+
Rational use of tools (pencil, spoon)	14+
Identification—animistic play (bear, doll)	13+
Dramatic play (doll's dinner)	24+

(8) *Pictures*

General (diffuse) interest in pictures	12+
Points to picture	14+
Identifies picture	18+
Imitates reading paper	14+

(9) *Language*

Babbling (vowels)	3+
Syllabic sounds	6–7
Jargon	12+
Using two words together	18
Sentence of three words	21–24
Calls himself by first name	21+
Pronouns	30

THE OBSERVATION OF QUALITY AND QUANTITY IN THE PSYCHOLOGICAL TESTING OF INFANTS

Marcelle Geber

PROFESSOR ARNOLD GESELL examined normal children and codified their development by stabilizing norms at 4 weeks, and every 4 weeks to 15 months, and then every 3 months to 24 months, and every 6 months up to 5 years. Through these norms it is possible to study, quantitatively, the development of the child in the four categories termed by Gesell: motor; adaptive; language; and personal-social. Before Gesell's test was introduced it was possible sometimes to get an impression of a certain backwardness, without being able to estimate its degree.

Backwardness may be due to psychogenic or organic causes, and sometimes, though there is no backwardness, the behaviour of the child is such that satisfactory quantitative results cannot be obtained.

The tester dealing with a very young child, must be persuasive in order to elicit a response from the child with his test material.

In view of the fact that, with the very young child, the results of the test depend essentially on the relationship established between the adult and the child, we must study in detail the behaviour of the child with the tester: it is of interest to the tester to see the child not only during the test but also before and after. Both the behaviour of the child and his attitude to the test, will be different according to whether the child is living in an institution or in his own family. For the sake of clarity I shall adopt the convention that the child is 'he' and the tester 'she'.

1. *In institutions.* What is the nature of the first contact? Sometimes a child accepts the adult easily. A very young child, not yet sitting up, allows himself to be picked up; he may or may not smile, but he does not seem to consider contact with an adult as being either pleasant or unpleasant. Sometimes the child clings to the adult and either seems to be at ease in the contact, or is frightened. Older children may walk towards the adult to try to attract her attention. Others refuse and turn away, but then may return and

play quite well; while yet others are completely indifferent to what is happening and allow themselves to be taken up just like bundles.

The experience of being left alone with an unknown adult in a strange room may be new to the child, for a young child is normally constantly in the company of someone he knows. What will he do when faced with the test objects, and what relationship will he establish with the tester?

(a) Sometimes the child does not use the tester at all, the toys are presented, he accepts and plays with them, and never turns towards the tester. However, if the latter deflects her attention a little from the child, he will no longer play with the toys, but may withdraw into himself or may turn towards her and convey the impression that he feels her presence, which he needs to continue the test—he needs to feel her interest. Sometimes he actively seeks the sympathy of the tester, turning towards her and smiling or talking, according to his age; he will touch her hands. Sometimes he needs to be encouraged by speech. Some children need practical help, e.g., being shown how to put the pellet into the bottle; others need physical contact and will not do anything until the tester adopts a more affectionate attitude.

Children may refuse test objects; sometimes they show frank opposition: they cry, scream, push away or dash to the ground the objects that are offered to them. Sometimes they are inhibited: they will not do anything but sit on the chair, and look at the adult or at the objects; later with restricted movements, as if, being unable to get rid of the adult, they may look as if they were trying to withdraw from the situation. Others lack all interest, remaining inert with a vague look in their eyes, with no interest in the adult, in the objects, or in the surrounding world.

The attitude taken towards the adult at the first contact does not allow one to predict the kind of relationship that the child will establish during the test.

(b) The behaviour towards objects is also connected with the relationship between child and tester. Some children are immediately and spontaneously interested in the objects submitted to them, and go ahead with the test in the way which is wanted. But very often the tester has to wait and must cultivate a permissive attitude, because sometimes ten or fifteen minutes will elapse before the child will do the test. At first he may simply play with the blocks, throw them on the floor or dash them against the table. Other children need the tester to be interested, with them, in the objects. Some refuse the objects: they either push them away or dash them down in active opposition, or do not take them because of inhibition. Some children are not interested in anything; these are the children who are like bundles in one's arms; and even if one sits for an hour, no results will be obtained. Inhibited children very often prefer small objects, and after fifteen minutes or so will decide to pick up a small object.

(c) There are qualitative differences in behaviour during test between institutional children and children in families. On the whole, institutional children will accept being in a strange room more easily than being with a stranger; some will not even look around the room and seem to be interested only in the adult. Other children will take an interest in the room, and the table, and will investigate everything. Others cry immediately, though they might accept the adult, and it is difficult to know whether this is because they are isolated with a stranger in a room or for some other reason.

The tester must know how to play with a child, how to speak or sing to the child. Sometimes the interview will begin very well and then, later, the child will dissolve into tears.

At the end of the test, the children who have not been interested in the adult will generally part from her quite easily, but others will cling to her and make it difficult to get them away. Others, perhaps the more intelligent ones, will continue to play with the objects, turning their backs on the adult. Some of the children will cry desperately when they leave the room, and in such a case things may be made easier if the child is allowed to take away one of the test objects.

The time taken by the test may be very variable; half-an-hour or much longer. Children who accept the adult easily do not use him during the test, which they accomplish rapidly, and leave without raising any difficulty. It is interesting to compare the attitude of the child towards the adult, the objects, and duration of his task, respectively. It is quite normal for younger children to be interested in the adult, and to take her into account, and this is a favourable sign. Institutionalized children pay less attention to what is going on around them; they are interested in the objects, and this is not a good sign, for the child who is more interested in objects than in adults is already tending to lose his contact with other persons.

2. *In the family.* One must take into account the behaviour of the child in his family. Many children of normal intelligence and favourable development, whose families are sound, will refuse the test,

unless the tester is well received by the mother. Some children need to turn towards their mother and even to be on the mother's lap; others, if they have a good relationship with their mother, will accept a stranger and co-operate with the tester.

Some mothers are themselves keenly interested in the proceedings, watch the child and encourage him, if he is not successful, with a smile or a word. Others are aggrieved and disappointed when they see the child fail in the test; others appear to lose interest and to ignore the situation, as if they cannot bear to see the child failing to do what they wish he could do.

Results. The results of the test must, of course, be integrated into the clinical context, because the Gesell test contains a large amount of material concerned with neuro-muscular development. Some children give incomplete results, as in the case of one little girl who accepted me with a smile; I took her into the test room. and, unexpectedly, she began to cry. It was impossible to console her. This child was in an institution because her mother was in hospital having another baby. The nurse said that her father came to see her in the room where I was to test her and perhaps she was disappointed that he was not there. Anyway, she did not want me to stay and was quite desolate.

Another child refused the test objects and violently pushed me away. The nurse told me that the child's mother had come to see her and had brought her a dress, which the child had refused to accept. The mother had insisted and had eventually gone away slamming the door. No doubt this scene with her mother affected the child's reception of the test.

Another little girl was in such a poor physical condition that she looked like a baby of 8 months rather than her real age, which was 2 years. There was some doubt as to whether she could or could not walk. Under test, she failed to do many of the things expected of her at her age. She sat hunched up on a small chair and refused to deal with any of the test objects. After trying in every possible way to obtain some response, I almost gave up after forty-five minutes, turned away and put the objects back into the box. She then climbed down from the chair and climbed up on to an adult's chair at the other end of the room, having walked to it by holding herself against the wall. The nurse would not believe this at first. This little girl improved so much under treatment that her development quotient, which at first was 30, is now 110.

To summarize: certain children do not make use of the adult when carrying out the test, and when this happens, care is called for because it is a danger signal and suggests that the child may be beginning to lose some of its potentiality for development. Some children ask for adult help, and others find the adult an encumbrance; either event is a sign of some contact and of potentiality for development. Some children are absolutely passive and refuse everything; the outlook for these children is serious. When a child is without interest in, or reason for, life, treatment is called for.

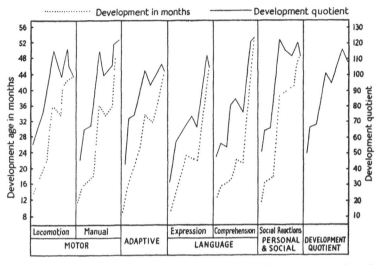

FIG. 1.—MARYSE Development tests between the ages of 2 years 1 month and 3 years 9 months.

In *Figure I* are shown the results of successive development tests of Maryse who, under treatment and with sound psychological handling, developed from a very backward condition to normality, in every sector of the test. It is of interest to note that Maryse apparently suffered a slight setback in the middle of the period, during which she temporarily lost ground in five of the six sectors. During this temporary phase, no doubt the clinical signs of regression would have been present.

Figure II shows graphically some of the effects of separation from their mothers, on children between the ages of 1 and 4 years. The group to which this graph relates comprised about fifty children in the same institution. During the first period, October, 1949–July, 1950, the institution remained as it had always been, but in the interval before the second period which began in October, 1950, certain alterations were made in the life of the children, partly as a result of the experience gained in the first period.

277

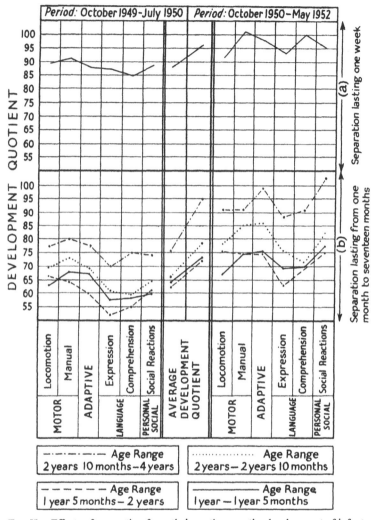

FIG. II.—Effects of separation from their mothers on the development of infants.

These alterations were in the direction of reducing the number of adults in contact with the children, giving children the opportunity of building up intimate, loving relationships with individual adults and increasing the environmental interest of their lives.

The upper Section (*a*) of Figure II relates to a group of children, aged from between 1 year and 1 year 5 months, who had been separated from their mothers for a period of one week, at the time of the test. During the earlier period the general level of development is low (average Development Quotient 88), but unfortunately it was not possible to test these children before separation, so that the significance of this fact cannot be assessed. In the later period, not only is the average Development Quotient higher, but the average in the various sectors of the development test are consistently higher —the two groups of children being comparable in all other respects.

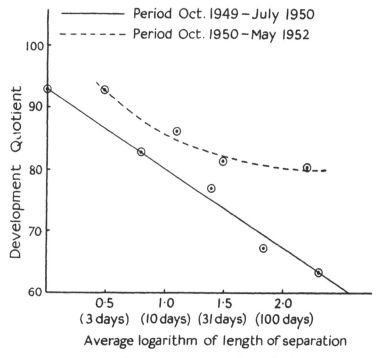

FIG. III.—The effect of protracted separation on development.

However, low levels of development in locomotion, language expression and social reactions are noticeable, all of these areas of development being of particular significance at the age of this group of children (1 year to 1 year 5 months).

The lower section (b) of Figure II relates to the effects of separation, lasting for more than thirty-two days, on children of four age groups from 1 to 4 years. In the earlier period, before alterations had been made in the life of the children, the low level of the Development Quotient is particularly striking. The average levels for the four groups, respectively, in the two periods are:

12–17 months: D.Q. 64; after improvements: 73
17–24 months: D.Q. 62; after improvements: 72
24–34 months: D.Q. 66; after improvements: 78
34–48 months: D.Q. 76; after improvements: 95

Generally speaking the younger the children, the greater the evidence of the harmful effects of separation, and the less can these be prevented by administrative devices. However, it will be seen that children between the ages of 1 year 5 months and 2 years were the worst affected.

From the shape of the curves it can be seen that locomotion and language were generally the most affected aspects of development, but that social reactions, greatly depressed in the earlier phase, appear to have responded favourably to the improvements in the institution.

Figure III indicates that, during the earlier period, the harmful effects of separation, on the child, were in a direct relationship with the duration of separation. After re-organization of the institution not only were the effects of separation less, but there was a tendency towards the condition becoming stabilized at a certain degree of backwardness.

Boys and girls appear, from these observations, to be about equally sensitive to separation from their mothers.

DISCUSSION

In Dr. Geber's experience, children in institutions behave differently to the tester from other children. This may be because they lack experience of human relationships. In general, they tend to cling to the tester and it is not easy to get them interested in the test objects. The difficulty can sometimes be overcome by facing the child immediately with the test objects without establishing any personal contact with him.

It is a good plan for the tester herself to fetch the child, and it often pays to carry him. If the child is busy with a toy, the tester should join in for a while, speak to him a little to attract his attention and then hold out her arms. If there is no response, the child should be picked up and carried to the room. In an institution, it is important to consider the nurses' feelings, and, for example, get them to attend to the child's wants rather than offend them by taking over complete charge.

Whether it is preferable to avoid having the child cling to the tester is arguable. Some testers advocate not establishing a personal contact but putting the child in contact with the equipment immediately. Against this is the view that the relationship of the child to the adult or the objects is a dynamic factor in the test.

It is also true that the results are not so good if the child clings to the tester, but the main interest of the test lies not so much in the quantitative result of the test as in the possibility of the child forming relationships with the adult. The effect of any such clinging is noted in the test record.

Two types of behaviour point, generally, to a rather low quotient: that of the child who makes no use of the adult, whether succeeding or failing in a test item; and that of the child who becomes interested in the test objects immediately, though in the latter case the test may be deceptively easy to administer.

It is easier to test a child in the family than in an institution. Without knowing the history of the development of the child, it is comparatively meaningless merely to know that he has a low development quotient. The quality is more important than the quantity.

Results tend to differ if the observer is changed. If the tester is neutral, the child's behaviour is dependent only on his own make-up, but during the test the tester is ready to respond to the child's needs, talking to the child, and, if necessary later, encouraging and helping the child. Patience is essential; hurry or worry in the tester tends to operate against optimum results.

It may be asked whether experience in institutions of playing with cubes and with similar objects, will influence the result of the tests; but, in fact, results are no better. In some families, children have toys of an educational nature, but this also appears to make no difference. It is wise, in the case of children in institutions, to begin with the cubes, because these seem to attract them; but with children in families to end with the cubes. The Gesell test material is that with which the child is accustomed to play; rattles and balls interest all children.

With institutional children, moreover, the cubes give the most reliable pointers; but if the child refuses the cubes, another object is tried and the cubes are given at the end of the test.

On the whole, children placed in foster-families, after having been in institutions, progress very much better than children in institutions, but one cannot put them into foster-homes until they have developed good contacts with adults.

The Gesell test has the advantage that it is concerned with both the neuromuscular and the psychological development of the child, therefore it allows of the ascertainment of both organic and psychogenic backwardness; but it cannot be assessed without some experience of normal reactions and without time to obtain proper results—perhaps half-an-hour or an hour at a time.

In clinics short of personnel it might be better to use less time-consuming and difficult tests for a rough sorting out of the children, and to reserve more elaborate investigations for the then known abnormal cases. The Gesell test is a sensitive and precise instrument for deep and subtle research, but only of limited application in a country with a shortage of psychological and medical personnel. The danger of the tests being given by other types of professional workers is that they, and even a nurse with special psychological training, would be in danger of over-looking an important neurological detail.

The idea that a paediatrician or general practitioner should be equipped with a technique to investigate how a child is developing, which would enable him to discover a slight deviation before sending the child to a psychiatrist or a paediatric hospital for further examination, is particularly attractive in areas where there is only one educational psychologist, fully occupied with testing school children.

Experience of teaching paediatricians the Gesell test in a course consisting of an hour's lecture per week for two months, has shown that very often, after going through the course, they still prefer to send the child to a more experienced person. They might get the quotient too low, either because they spent only a short time giving the test, or were not sufficiently permissive and did not let the child make full use of what they gave it. The most difficult thing to learn is the right attitude, and this only comes with much experience in psychological practice.

EDUCATIONAL SYMPOSIUM: TECHNIQUES AND METHODS OF PRESENTATION

Alan Staniland

I SHALL TRY to give a general idea of the types of apparatus available for education by visual methods, and to say something of the attitude one should have towards these methods.

While I shall limit myself to types of projection other than cinematography, it is worth mentioning that there is one very valuable form of cinematographic projection which we did not see at the Seminar—the moving diagrammatic film.

The projection of still pictures is of particular interest to anyone who must experiment on a cheaper scale than with the cine film. There are three main types, each of which has certain advantages. The first is the *episcope*, which is unique because it is the only projector which will show pictures not specially prepared for projection. It will show illustrations from books, picture-postcards, and especially coloured illustrations or diagrams. The episcope is the least efficient and most cumbersome of all the still-picture projectors, but it is specially useful with material drawn from many sources, that is not worth the expense of permanent photographic record.

The old *standard lantern*, like the episcope, is often rather a cumbersome instrument, but small types of this lantern are available which are efficient and very easily portable, and adequate for all but large lecture audiences. The size of the slides varies between 3¼ in. sq. (8¼ cm.) in England and up to 12 × 9 cm. in Germany and some other parts of Europe.

Waterproof drawing-ink on non-waterproof cellophane lends itself to easy tracing, and the cellophane slides are projected by putting them between thin glass carriers. They save a great deal of labour. They are especially suitable for more complicated drawings than can be made with chalk in the course of a lecture.

One other kind of hand-made slide is worth mention, namely, sketching on a glass plate prepared with a mixture of shellac and lampblack (fine carbon). A graph or basic diagram of any type can be thrown on to a blackboard and can be used as a basis on which to work with chalk.

The third kind of projector is the *miniature lantern* which was

283

originally designed to show the smaller photographs produced by miniature cameras—pictures $1\frac{1}{4}$ in $\times$ 1 in., or 36 $\times$ 24 mm. in size. Either black and white or colour pictures can be shown very well by this type of projector. The slides are quite easy and cheap to produce, but it is difficult to produce hand-made slides on a base measuring only $1\frac{1}{2} \times$ 1 in., so that practically all material requires a photographic process of some kind. But such miniature slides, as well as being projected individually, can be put into the lantern on a length of film, which may take as many as a hundred small slides joined together, with a projector designed to change the picture by a turn of a knob; in other words, a *film-strip*. A strip of a hundred pictures can be kept in a small tin and posted without risk of breakage. It is the cheapest form of photographic projection available, costing, say, only $4\frac{1}{4}$d. to 6d. as against four or five times that amount for the photographic lantern slide.

The film-strip has developed some interesting possibilities; it shows a sequence of pictures and within limits can be turned forwards and backwards. At its best it needs to be designed very much as a cinema film though on a smaller scale; but because it is fairly cheap the sequence can be used to multiply the number of pictures and to show several pictures related in a certain order.

In my work of training and encouraging teachers in the use of illustration, during the last five years, I have made a habit of asking at the beginning of each year how many students think they can draw. Usually the proportion is about 5 per cent. Working on the other 95 per cent has made me aware of something which I can only call 'visual illiteracy'. I could give some amusing examples of students' drawings in which the essential fault is not manual, but perceptual. In children's drawings, the drawings and the knowledge keep in step, but somewhere in adolescence they seem to get out of step. The inability of these young adults to draw was due to failure to see objects in their proper relation to each other.

In illustrating subject matter that requires special knowledge, it is particularly important that the expert should be able to conceive and initiate, even if the professional artist must be called in to complete the job. The best way of describing the initial attitude that is most favourable, is as an attempt to see the problem as a child might see it, broken up into articulated parts.

The aesthetic qualities of the material not only make it pleasant to look at, but may directly arouse the essential response that is needed. Emotion is an indication of interest, but interest is only firmly established when we can join with it technical curiosity. The commercial artist can often give the aesthetic finish, but clarity of conception is the job of the expert.

EDUCATIONAL SYMPOSIUM:
THE PROCESS OF COMMUNICATION

G. P. Meredith

THERE IS a story that goes around the British Army about a message that was sent down a line of soldiers in a trench during a battle: 'Send up reinforcements, we are going to advance'. By the time the message had passed through twenty or thirty different persons and reached the other end of the line it had become, 'Lend the Major fourpence, he's going to a dance.'

There are many possible causes of failure of communication, but we do not always recognize them, except when a wire breaks or a letter fails to be delivered. Those who have to spend any part of their lives communicating or educating have a duty to be aware of all the many ways in which communications can fail, which means, to think as seriously about this process and in just as technical a way as the electrician has to think about a telephone line.

If the amount of time we spend in purely physical contact with people, either manipulating their bodies or operating on them, or giving them medicine or injections, is compared with the amount of time we spend talking and writing to people, showing things to them or organizing for other people to do those things, it will be realized that first and foremost we are mental communicators far more than physical manipulators. Since we spend so much time communicating, and what we have to communicate is of so much importance, it is worth analysing the process of communication and its technique.

The first principle we might consider is that all interaction between persons is an act of communication. Secondly, every act of communication involves six elements: 1, the communicator; 2, a field of meaning, the kind of facts which have to be communicated, perhaps about feeding or disease or babies; 3, the message referring to that field; 4, the 'language' in which the message is communicated, whether it be speech, pictures, diagrams, mathematical symbols, and so on; 5, the medium or apparatus of communication, such as a lantern slide, or simply the human voice, the air and the ear of the listener; and 6, the recipient, the person for whom all this is intended. The recipient is the most important factor, because without him there would be no point in communicating.

What is the relation between the communicator and the other five elements? Obviously the communicator must be well informed about the field of meaning. Some people think that is enough. But all of us have had experience of experts, talking about their subjects, who quite fail to communicate. They were experts in the subject, but not in communication. Next, the communicator needs to be able to formulate the message; in other words, to extricate from his detailed grasp of the facts a suitable message for communication. You can never communicate everything about any fact; there must always be an act of selection in communication.

Then the communicator has to translate the content of his message into language. It would be naive to think of any act of communication as a direct relationship between the speaker and hearer, though we take for granted all those intervening processes because they have become automatized. It is when communication fails us that we become aware of the complexity of those processes.

In considering the recipient himself, we need to bear in mind our knowledge of the varied kinds of perception, and the influences on perception of all sorts of physical, social, emotional and other factors. Even if all our processes of communication were technically perfect there must still be a failure in those cases in which the mind of the recipient is such that it cannot take in the message in the form in which it is given. The communicator needs, in relation to the recipient, not only a knowledge of the latter's objective needs—what information he has to supply—but also an ability to project himself into the mind of the recipient and influence his readiness and aptitude for the message.

I would stress the need for the imaginative capacity of the communicator to build up in his own mind an understanding of the mind of the recipient, taking into account what he knows about the latter's habit of speech and intellectual background, and all the other information which may tell about his mind. The communicator must then think about the message and the language of the message in relation to the readiness of the recipient's mind to receive it.

Part Eight

SUMMING-UP

SUMMING-UP

Kenneth Soddy

THERE CAN BE no clear-cut non-statistical method by which a Seminar such as that at Chichester can be evaluated, and indeed the criteria of success must necessarily depend upon the expectations of the organizers and of all who took part. Inevitably there must be multiple aims for such an undertaking and in the case of the Chichester Seminar, those of promoting international understanding, promoting technical and professional education, exchanging information on modern advances in the child development field, and promoting mental hygiene projects on a world-wide scale, can be mentioned. Perhaps the best way of indicating to the reader some of the effects, on the Faculty and participants, of attending the Seminar, is to give a short account of what the people present actually felt about it at the time. Whether these feelings can be held to justify the enormous expenditure of effort and money which the Seminar entailed, must then be left to others to judge. Certainly it can be said that no one who was present had any doubt that the Seminar was eminently well worth-while.

Participants' own opinions. Some two days before the end of the Seminar a short questionnaire was distributed to Faculty and participants alike. Everyone was asked to state what he had hoped to gain from the Seminar, what he had actually expected to gain, and what he thought the actual gain had been. All were also invited to make comments and criticisms; and the most general of these was that it would have been better if the questionnaire had been distributed on the last day, because so much had happened, in the last two days, to clarify outstanding issues and to give those who were present a deep sense of satisfaction in what they had experienced. The result of the questionnaire was remarkable in that there was a 100 per cent return.

Replies to the first two questions varied between two extremes. Some had absolutely no idea what to expect, because they had had no information, and others had hoped or expected to gain a whole armoury of weapons to help them in their work. One lady evidently had a low level of expectation because, as she baldly stated, she was a Government servant and had come because she had been sent.

U   289

Perhaps the majority had felt uncertain about what was to happen, but many had hoped to gain specific factual information which would be of use to them in their work. Quite a few had clear-cut and realistic expectations, looking forward to a general reorientation; whilst some, quite frankly, were looking for comfort and friends, and for antidotes to national or professional isolation. The replies can best be illustrated by extracts from the participants' own words. First, the uncertainty with which the majority approached the Seminar: 'It is difficult to say what I had expected of the Seminar, because I just left all possibilities open'; and, again: 'I had little advance notice and it was impossible to have well formulated ideas before arrival.' Someone from a remote and backward country explained that he had never heard of any Mental Health organizations. Another participant was astonished to find that the Seminar was inter-disciplinary: she had expected to find only social workers present; she was, however, delighted with what she found. Doubts about the nature of international group-work led one member to approach the Seminar with an open mind and it was, no doubt, a similar feeling which prompted another to say: 'I had no clear idea about what I expected, so do not know if I have got it.'

A sense of personal insufficiency pervaded some of the participants' replies: 'I felt a sense of trepidation at the prospect of associating with people who know so much more about infant psychology than I do.' 'I feared to come across an exclusively dynamic or deterministic point of view and an attempt to determine norms for everybody.' One participant was greatly impressed by the notion that human behaviour, individual and in groups, can be subjected to scientific study: he wrote 'I was rather perplexed that, after two great wars, our life has become more and more restricted on all sides by controls, rations, permits and licences. I thought that the recurrent cycle of violence and destruction was largely due to the fact that man's understanding and control over physical nature has far outrun his control over human nature.'

As for the more clear-cut expectations: 'I expected, and I actually found, data concerning various cultures, stand-points and reactions different from my own and because of this have undergone an evolution and change in my own opinions . . . ' A typical need was 'to learn from other countries how they were developing their mental health programme' and there was a recurrent theme, in the replies, of expecting to have personal discussion with other people engaged with similar problems in different countries, and to study cultural factors.

Many expectations were concerned with the gaining of specific information, the keeping in touch with modern thought and trends and the meeting with well-known people. One participant wanted: 'Suggestions or direct answers to some of the many problems we are all faced with, such as therapy and preventive problems; measures to solve problems of crippled children, deaf and dumb, blind, feeble-minded, and delinquent children.' Someone wanted more precise knowledge about hospitalization and young infants, and the later effects of separation in early infancy, placement in observation centres, and so on. There was a call for facts, figures and statistics concerning infant development, well epitomised by: 'I expected to find what it takes to make the thing go. I hoped that a set of general rules, educational advice, and a list of errors and mistakes to be avoided in the field of child-rearing, would be drawn up from this series of lectures and discussions.'

Many participants came with a sense of isolation. One wrote: 'What I hoped to get, among other things, was comfortable accommodation and friends.' The lone worker eagerly embraced this opportunity of learning new ideas of mental hygiene development after twenty years of personal work. The isolation of many countries and the isolation of many professional people in unsympathetic communities, particularly in widely scattered populations, served to heighten the expectation of participants. This was particularly strongly felt in countries where literature in the mother-tongue is restricted and where there is no great aptitude for reading in other languages. Interprofessional co-operation was another strong motive, particularly among these lonely people.

Participants' own account of their gains. On the whole the response was very gratifying to the organizers. Nearly everyone found friendship and an enhanced international understanding, a widening of horizons and a great stimulation and inspiration for their work. The majority also found enrichment in the area of higher technical education.

The most important gain of all was a new sense of orientation. It was a relief for some to find that the mental health movement was not so much an innovation as an orientation, and properly part of the task of all engaged in medical and social welfare work. Many were stimulated by renewing contact with the phenomena of child development, especially through the films; some had never been familiar with the developing child. 'The method of work was far different from what I was accustomed to and this represented an enriching experience.' One participant gained some new basic points of view and a new kind of approach: 'Throughout we got a sense of widening horizons.'

Perhaps the most striking new experience for most people was an introduction to an anthropological point of view: 'The comparison of the problems of different countries and the contributions of the anthropologist have stimulated me to think about our own problems in a new way.' The Seminar was felt as a stimulus to further study and the group-work, the allowing for emotional reactions of the participants, was an eye-opener for many. Over and over again participants expressed a sense of disappointment that they had not obtained more concrete information, but added that, in spite of this, they had undergone a clarification of concepts and an understanding of human and cultural relationships. Cultural pattern and the background of the cases were indeed a surprise to many; but no more than the immense amount of detail with which the case histories of these young children had been presented. An introduction to other ideas was experienced by one participant, who wrote: 'Lectures, group discussions and interpersonal contacts represented for me a "bath" in mental hygiene and helped me to reconsider the whole problem in the light of ideas I had tended to discard because they are not widely accepted by the school of psychiatric training to which I belong.' One participant did not learn anything new but suffered a flux of thinking 'which may lead me to abandon the fruitless organicist position.'

As well as general orientation there were more practical gleanings: 'The Seminar has given an impetus to the family fostering of young infants; it will reduce the referrals to institutions and improve the functioning of institutions which remain.' 'I have also thought of ways in which we can in our public hospitals revise our regulations for the visiting of parents, the stay of children in hospitals and a few other ideas which can be carried out.' If this participant succeeds in this, the Seminar will have been worth-while for this alone.

Knowledge gained was deemed to be of value in teaching, and in practical work in a school Mental Hygiene Service. 'I hope I can introduce what I have learnt to my own circle.' The importance of the good mother-child relationship was vivid and real to many participants, who went away determined to introduce these principles into their day-to-day practical management. A participant came to realize that there was more than one way of doing good work: 'If anything emerges clearly from all the discussions, it is that the love-life of the child, his adjustment to filial and fraternal relationships in the family, may well set the general pattern for all later social, vocational, and marital adjustments.' There was also realization of the need to consider the family as a whole in its social, cultural, and economic life in society and to consider the consequences of the familial environment on the day-to-day habits and the psycho-physical development of a child.

As in the case of the first question, there were many participants with a sense of personal incompetence: many expressed astonishment at the range of ideas considered important. One, from a backward country, questioned for the first time the wisdom of copying the more advanced countries, in the developing life of his own community. A sense of personal development was experienced: 'I have got very few concrete instructions useful to me when I return home. At first I felt this as a considerable disappointment, but as time went on I realized that I was getting something, which to me personally, and with regard to my ability to handle problems in my daily work and in my relationship to different groups of people, was more valuable than facts and concrete instruction.'

The human need for friendship was well catered for and many wished the Seminar to last a great deal longer because of this. 'I feel most grateful and pleased for the agreeable and pleasant way in which all arrangements have been made, for the gay and informal spirit which the leaders of the Seminar have given to our time together and for the many interesting personal contacts . . .' The happiness of the experience is referred to again and again: 'after the initial anxiety . . . I began to feel that, at enormous effort and expense, many important people had been brought together to tell us much which, through our experience and our reading, we already knew. This feeling quickly passed and I began to see that the experience gained in my personal and working life must be systematized and based on specific observation if I was to use it in influencing attitudes towards the care and needs of the young child and towards the meaning of mental health. I am really grateful to the World Federation for Mental Health for all I have acquired.'

International understanding. International understanding was a preoccupation of a great many. On the one hand the opportunity to 'satisfy certain false doubts in the mind of many delegates and to give them the real facts is certainly one of the most active ways towards a better mutual understanding.' One participant wrote: 'Best of all, I realized international understanding and sympathy. It seems to me that the whole world is after all just a big family.' Professional people were keen to take the opportunity to compare their ideas with their opposite numbers in different countries: some discovered that they liked people of other nationalities better than they had thought. 'One need not despair that International Conferences are futile, we can learn much from each other's mistakes, where the cultural levels are comparable.'

The 'splendid isolation' of some professional workers, particularly among the medical disciplines, was commented on unfavourably and the opportunity was welcomed for discussion of case problems with professional colleagues from another discipline. However, the individual stimulation of discussing ideas with people brought up in a different culture is not without its stresses; and whereas most people wanted the Seminar to go on for a good deal longer, a minority thought that ten days was quite long enough and that longer constituted a strain. In spite of this, the majority would echo the remark of one of our number: 'from my personal standpoint the Seminar was a signal success, I got what I had hoped to get.'

Criticisms and suggestions. There was a general feeling that much remained to be done and that the case material had not been used exhaustively enough. This was combined with a hope that another Seminar could be held in from two to four years' time, with the same people if possible; and some fostered the ambition to establish more permanent study groups in various countries. Such suggestions, as all who are experienced in the international field have discovered, are virtually impossible to carry out.

There was a feeling that the terminology was confused and confusing and that better progress would have been made by more consideration of general principles in mental health, first. Some people thought that not enough practical application had been indicated, and that the discussion had, on the whole, departed too far from the lectures; but, in the main, group sessions were extremely popular and their lack of rigid form was much enjoyed.

It is worth noting that many people felt that a useful contribution could have been made by holding supplementary discussions of groups made up of one profession. Groups of this sort might have reported back to the whole Seminar for further inter-disciplinary discussion.

Conclusion. The experience of being present at the Seminar and of reading these comments has left behind an abiding impression of a quite extraordinary degree of enlargement of horizon and of a high quality of friendship. On the level of human contact alone and of international understanding, the Seminar would have been worthwhile. But there was much more than this, there was an unexpected amount of detailed information contained in the material placed before the Seminar. There was far more factual material of child development gathered together than is customarily found in any such teaching programme. Writing for myself, I was brought up against the fact that the child is a developing organism, with much greater clarity than ever before. We realized that more might have been done had case material been available at an earlier date and had

294

it been possible to lay the plans, say, six months earlier throughout. However, these case materials remain and will repay further and repeated study. I am convinced of the value of the free group discussion method, provided that there is time enough for the members of the groups to get to know each other; and I am convinced of the value of inter-disciplinary, inter-professional, international groups provided that there is no pressure to create a factual report.

Most of us gained a clearer realization of the degree to which we are embedded in our own cultural pattern; and we learnt much of what appertains to the organization of such international occasions. It is hoped that sufficient experience was gained for participants themselves to organize teaching seminars in their own communities. Perhaps at this Seminar we did not find a final answer to the difficulties involved in conducting a full seminar discussion on a lecture, nor deal successfully with the handicaps inherent in the technique of simultaneous interpretation. More thought and experiment need to be given to these problems.

Dr. Aubry remarked in the closing session, in extension of a thought of Dr. Margaret Mead's, that it is important for people at a seminar, like children in a culture of change, to be capable of building a nest in a storm; but at the Chichester Seminar there had been no storm and international tensions had not arisen. The Seminar had triumphantly demonstrated the principle of international and inter-disciplinary team work. Dr. Margaret Mead herself, in the same session, concluded that one of the purposes of the Seminar had been to learn what a seminar was like. We had erred in not realizing that our members would not be called upon to give and receive in equal degree; but we had at least succeeded in maintaining spontaneous interest and had had real discussion in the groups. Professor MacCalman thought that the Seminar had been a miracle of concord and good human relationships and that the participants would return to their own communities with renewed belief that of the three virtues, faith, hope and charity, the greatest was charity. I can do no better than to close this account with his further thought that participants had learnt that they could love their neighbours and could be found lovable, that they had learnt to accept as well as give affection. This was an enriching experience.

> Happy to meet,
> Hoping to meet again,
> Sorry to part,
> Bon Accord!

FILM REFERENCES

All films are 16 mm.

BATESON, Gregory, and MEAD, Margaret.

A Balinese Family. 2 reels. 22 minutes. Silent. Margaret Mead, American Museum of Natural History, Central Park West at 79th Street, New York.

Bathing Babies in Three Cultures. 1 reel. 11 minutes. Silent. (As above.)

First Days in the Life of a New Guinea Baby. 2 reels. 22 minutes. Silent. (As above.)

Childhood Rivalry in Bali and New Guinea. 2 reels. 22 minutes. Silent. (As above.)

Dance and Trance in Bali. 2 reels. 22 minutes. Silent. (As above.)

Karba's First Years. (As above.)

JOSELIN, Arnold G.

Life Begins in Leeds. 5 reels. 50 minutes. Sound. World Federation for Mental Health, 19 Manchester Street, London, W.1., and Leeds University, U.K.

ROBERTSON, James.

A Two-Year-Old Goes to Hospital. 4 reels. 60 minutes. Sound. Tavistock Clinic, 2 Beaumont Street, London, W.1.

ROUDINESCO (AUBRY), Jenny.

Monique (Maternal Deprivation in Young Children). 2 reels. 22 minutes. Sound. J. Aubry, Association pour la Santé Mentale de l'Enfance, 40 rue François I, Paris VIII.

SPITZ, René, and WOLF, Katherine A.

Grief—A Peril in Infancy. 3 reels. 35 minutes. Silent. René Spitz, 1150 Fifth Avenue, New York 28.

Mother-Child Relations. 2 reels. 22 minutes. Silent. (As above.)

The Smiling Response. Silent. (As above.)

STONE, L. Joseph.

A Backward Look at Abbey's First Two Years. 4 reels. 60 minutes. New York University Film Library.

BIBLIOGRAPHY

(1) BAIN, Katherine. 'The Incidence of Breast-feeding in Hospitals in the United States.' *Pediatrics*, Vol. II, No. 3, 1948.

(2) BOWLBY, John. 'Maternal Care and Mental Health.' WHO Technical Monograph Series, No. 2, Geneva, 1951.
Also in abridged version 'Child Care and the Growth of Love.' Penguin Books, London, 1953.

(3) BOWLBY, J., ROBERTSON, J., and ROSENBLUTH, D. 'A Two-Year-Old Goes to Hospital.' *Psycho-analytic Study of the Child*, 7, 82–94. 1952.

(4) BRUNET O. and LEZINE, I. 'Le développement psychologique de la première enfance.' P.U.F., Paris, 1951.

(5) BURLINGHAM, Dorothy, and FREUD, Anna. 'Infants without Families.' Allen & Unwin, London, 1943.

(6) BURLINGHAM, Dorothy, and FREUD, Anna. 'Young Children in Wartime.' Allen & Unwin, London, 1942.

(7) Children's Bureau, 'INFANT CARE'. U.S. Federal Security Agency, 1951.

(8) Department of Health for Scotland. 'Health of the Mother and Child.' (Distributor: Central Council for Health Education.)

(9) ERIKSON, Eric. 'Childhood and Society.' Imago Publishing Co., London, 1951.

(10) FREUD, Anna, and DANN, Sophie. 'Experiment in Group Up-bringing.' *Psychoanalytic Study of the Child*, Vol. VI, 1951.

(11) GESELL, A., and THOMPSON, H. 'THE PSYCHOLOGY OF EARLY GROWTH'. Macmillan. New York, 1938.

(12) GIBBON, Lewis Grassic, and MACDIARMID, Hugh. 'SCOTTISH SCENE'. pp. 117–18. Jarrolds Ltd., London, 1934.

(13) GILLILAND, A. R. 'Environmental Influence on Infant Intelligence Test Scores.' *Harvard Educational Revue*, No. 19, 1949.

(14) GOLDFARB, W. 'The Effects of Early Institutional Care on Adolescent Personality.' *Journal of Experimental Education*, No. 12, 1943.

(15) KLATSKIN, E. H. 'Intelligence Test Performance at One Year among Infants raised with Flexible Methodology.' *Journal of Clinical Psychology*, Vol. VIII, No. 3, 1952.

(16) LORENZ, K. 'Der Kumpan in der Umwelt des Vogels.' *J. Ornithol.* No. 83, 1935. (Abridged and translated into English, Auk, No. 54, pp. 245–273.)

(17) LORENZ, K. 'King Solomon's Ring.' Methuen, London, 1952.

(18) MEAD, Margaret, *ed.* 'Cultural Patterns and Technical Change.' Manual prepared by WFMH. Published by UNESCO. Tensions and Technology Series, Paris, 1953.

(19) MEREDITH, H. V. 'Physical Growth from Birth to Two Years: I. Stature, *University of Iowa Studies in Child and Welfare,* No. 19, 1943.

(20) OGBURN, W. F. 'Social Change.' New York, 1922.

(21) PEATMAN, J. G. and HIGGONS, R. A. 'Development of Sitting, Standing, and Walking of Children reared with Optimal Pediatric Care.' *American Journal of Orthopsychiatry,* No. 10, London, 1933.

(22) READ, Grantly Dick. 'Childbirth Without Fear.' Heinemann, London, 1933.

(23) ROBERTS, CORNER and DAVIES. 'Textbook for Health Visitors.' Bailliere, Tindall & Cox, London, 1951.

(24) ROBERTSON, J. 'Some Responses of Young Children to the Loss of Maternal Care.' *Nursing Times,* April, 1953.

(25) SCOTT, J. P. 'Social Behaviour, Organization and Leadership in a Small Flock of Domestic Sheep.' *Comp. Psychol. Monog.* 18, No. 4, 1945.

(26) SPOCK, Ben. 'Pocket Book of Baby and Child Care.' Pocket Books Inc., Rockefeller Centre, New York, 1946.

Addendum

(27) KOFFKA, K. 'Principles of Gestalt Psychology.' Routledge and Kegan Paul, London, 1935.

INDEX

304